Psychiatry Made Simple

Dr. Pete's Guide to Your Mental Health

PETER J. LITWIN, MD

authorHOUSE®

AuthorHouse™
1663 Liberty Drive
Bloomington, IN 47403
www.authorhouse.com
Phone: 1-800-839-8640

Published by AuthorHouse   12/22/2014

ISBN: 978-1-4969-6000-9 (sc)
ISBN: 978-1-4969-5996-6 (e)

Contents

About the Author

Dr. Pete is a seasoned and caring professional with twenty-four years of experience treating a wide range of psychiatric conditions, from neurosis to psychosis, from mania to catatonia. He writes about his varied experiences in an informal, easily accessible style that sheds light on the confusing field of behavioral health. How do we separate "different" or unusual behavior from true disorders? Why do people suffer from so much stress these days, in spite of our high standard of living and our access to effective treatments? How does a psychiatrist choose between Zoloft and Wellbutrin? Does psychiatric illness result mostly from our genes or our genesis? And why do most people make such irrational decisions? We seem to choose quite poorly—jobs we resent, spouses we divorce, homes we try to sell two years after moving into them, doctors who try to help us but only get two visits to do so before they are dismissed.

Dr. Pete offers a stimulating discussion of all these topics and more in this guide to our mental health. He views his work as preventive in that he strives to motivate patients to care for themselves emotionally, physically, medically, financially, and spiritually. He also attempts to move patients away from an overly responsible and anxious mode, to a focus on rewarding and health-minded behavior. In fact he hopes to set an example for his patients by cycling to his office, spending time on the beach or in his sailboat, relaxing in his wildflower garden and —most important—reflecting on how to improve as a healer. He resides on the Jersey Shore with his family and is often found reading or writing in various parts of the house.

Introduction

Why Does Psychiatry Matter?

Consider the following three extremely different scenarios:

> "I knew she was the one when she walked into the Italian restaurant I used to eat at every Sunday. You should've seen the way she ate those mussels—she never left a drop of broth behind. We were married three months later, and now it's been forty-five years. I never even looked at another woman."

> "I can't believe what he did. We were together for eight years, and he always talked about tying the knot. Then he suddenly moved out last year. Just last week I heard he's engaged to some girl he met in that Italian place. I did everything for him. How could he do this to me?"

> "I went to see this real shark of a divorce attorney last week. I caught my wife texting some yoga instructor. I can't believe she would do this to me. I haven't been around much, what with my work and my fishing trips and golf outings at the club, but that shouldn't make any difference."

These are all different patients' actual stories, which they have revealed to me over the years. You can see how much latitude there can be in the decision to marry or to end a marriage. So, even though my chosen field will never be able to predict who marries whom and certainly not whose marriage lasts and whose ends up in divorce court, you can't blame us psychiatrists, psychologists, therapists, and marriage counselors for trying. We are indeed fortunate to have the opportunity to gain the trust of our patients, who include us in their most difficult and complex decisions. As a medically trained clinician who appreciates the tremendous role of our genetic input, as well as our temperament, our traits, and our development, I have prized this access to my patients' inner lives. I certainly appreciate my colleagues who treat life-threatening disorders and help regulate their patients' physiology, but I view my own work as a more perplexing but ever-rewarding enterprise, in which my goals are the same as my patients'—maximizing their ability to pursue happiness and reach their full potential.

But what's it all about? Why choose psychiatry?

As a student I became more and more committed to the process of understanding human behavior to the best of my ability. The actual practice of psychiatry has reminded me on a daily basis of my own limited grasp of the field. Not a single day passes without moments of surprise, concern, or even bafflement. My patients continue to defy my theories and to teach me much more than the professors from my residency training program. This book is designed to help provide the foundation, from a practical and real-world perspective, that will help you, the reader, feel more comfortable in this area in which most of the terrain remains uncharted. I also hope to clarify some of the confusion which may result from the use of technical terms that you might come across in many settings, including the media, everyday conversation, the Internet, and various health care facilities. To my knowledge there is no layperson's guide to many of these issues that explains these concepts and sheds light on a critical and relevant area in our society. Even more critical is the fact that, in spite of our efforts and progress in the field of psychiatry over the past hundred years, many well-designed studies have demonstrated that our citizens are more likely to suffer from a mood or anxiety disorder in the twenty-first century than in times past. All the more reason, then, that we need to be able to identify, with a reasonable degree of confidence, when a given individual might be suffering from a significant form of mental illness and how to go about understanding and addressing this problem. Though I do not view this book as a self-help guide, at least the reader will have some idea of where to start in his or her own appreciation of mental health and how to take care of him- or herself more effectively.

As a practicing psychiatrist who presumably could have entered whichever branch of medicine I wished, I have often faced questions about my chosen field. "What made you go into psychiatry?" is a common query, posed by various skeptical souls who clearly do not feel that this line of work represents the true practice of medicine. Or perhaps they are implying that this field does not adequately challenge my intellect or skill set. Or, alternatively, that my work is futile, since they are certain that my patients do not ever really get "cured," no matter how we define that term.

Well, since my days in preschool, I have always sought out a challenge—at times, to my detriment—rather than take the easy way out. And there is plainly no area of study more complex, unpredictable, surprising, irrational, and perplexing than everyday human behavior. We all know that there are many—in reality, countless—mysteries to be discovered in other medical specialties and scientific fields, but the question of what is going through any given person's mind at any given moment is also a mystery. Ultimately, what makes someone tick from a behavioral perspective will—at least in my opinion—never be fully explained. By definition, as our patron, Freud, pointed out, the motivation for human behavior is multifactorial rather than simple. This means that each action we take results from a series of inputs, which all are weighed and evaluated in what we call the executive center of the brain. After consideration, which might require milliseconds (a major league player swinging his bat) or possibly decades (a confirmed bachelor finally deciding to pop the question), the person makes a decision. A considerable range of reactions and time frames factor into this process. There might be few inputs, as, for example, when you touch a hot piece of pizza and drop it, or many, as in choosing a career or a partner. The former action is conscious, in that we would all agree that the pizza was hot. The latter decision, however, can often be quite cryptic in that we actually make difficult choices largely based on the way we are programmed. In reality we have a multitude of unconscious reactions which we might not be aware of which are powerful influences in the course of our lives.

Chapter 1

Why Does Mental Illness Exist?

Are your patients actually sick or just exaggerated versions of "normal" individuals?

Perhaps this seems like a silly question that will lead only to some protracted and ultimately irrelevant discussion. Many thinkers have viewed mental disorders as a reaction to, or construct of, our society, rather than true illnesses. In other words, when we are unable to adapt to an impossible set of demands, we develop a syndrome that reflects our state of frustration and disenfranchisement. Most of us would certainly recognize our society's role in the increasing incidence of stress-based conditions. This can take one of two forms, or a combination of both. In the first, which generally occurs in totalitarian and intolerant regimens, the community as a whole—or the powers that be—label culturally or politically unacceptable behavior as mental illness. In the second process, society exerts stress on its citizens, some of whom will respond by developing mental illness. However, my goal is not to indict our society or culture as oppressive or intolerant but instead to underscore the impact of the enormous pressures that we all face, largely due to the complexity of modern life. This point is reflected in the fact that all societies—regardless of their political or cultural underpinnings—generally exhibit the same rate of mental illness.

But most of your patients don't have such a tough life—why can't they see how much worse things could be?

This is a common misconception which many patients come up against. We speak of patients as the "worried well." Many of my colleagues in medicine refer to the majority of outpatients as "neurotic." Though this label has some value in that neurosis can be a useful term in identifying patients who are suffering from internal or intrapsychic conflicts, this is like referring to the average cardiac patient as a constellation of partially clogged arteries. Once the patient comes into our office presenting a past history of myocardial infarction, the medical term for a heart attack, we tend to take them much more seriously. In the same vein, we often sit up and pay more attention to a patient who we know has been floridly manic or psychotic. Those latter states are generally associated with dramatic and easily recognizable disorders, with clear symptoms and biological underpinnings. The more common outpatient, who often presents a long pattern of anxiety and frustration, can be (on the surface, at least) less rewarding in some perspectives. We might view them as overreacting to a fairly trivial set of issues, or we might view their discontent as a form of simply expecting or wanting the world to be different than the reality. So, in some fairly primitive models, the neurotic patient has failed to mature for a variety of reasons and is not able to adapt successfully to his or her circumstances. In other words, such patients are fixated, or caught in an earlier stage of development. Those who accept that life is not always fair and that we have the obligation to expect and adapt to some setbacks and frustration will in the long term have much less need for my services.

I never promised you a rose garden!

We appear, however, to live in the midst of an epidemic of anxiety, angst, frustration, anger, and resentment. Many patients—or more accurately, we, as a society—struggle with a sense of injustice, of being cheated in some way. Our expectations somehow set us up for a negative outcome, just as a football fan who loudly proclaims that his or her team is the best in the division might be forced to eat crow at the end of the season should his or her team fail to make the play-offs. Our expectations largely dictate how we react to the world and whether we achieve a sense of happiness or peace. Unfortunately, for most of us, modifying our expectations can be just as difficult as reducing our cholesterol or our blood pressure. In fact, we are programmed to a large extent with these expectations, just as a young person generally develops strong religious or political beliefs, which then become quite entrenched and difficult to challenge.

But Doctor Pete, I have no reason to be so miserable. It doesn't make sense.

In my experience many of my patients ask themselves why they can't be grateful for what they have and why they would find themselves depressed or anxious, given the fact that they generally have what they need. Often there is an acute sense of guilt for somehow failing to appreciate their families, their jobs, their homes, their friends, and their possessions. Even though, as citizens of developed countries in the twenty-first century, we possess more material wealth and more access to various forms of support, mental illness has in fact affected more and more of our citizens. While we no longer face adversity such as saber-toothed tigers, the black plague, or ice ages, we nevertheless confront various unseen threats and dangers on a daily basis. We face volatility everywhere we look—in our faltering economy, more and more frequent rounds of layoffs, the bewildering swings of the stock market, our unstable climate, the rising rate of divorce, the increasing mobility and resulting sense of rootlessness of the extended family. A society that presents so much change and flux, one that offers almost limitless potential for success and growth, also provides us with a multitude of opportunities to flounder and fail. Many individuals who find the workforce or the social network difficult to navigate—often through no fault of their own—eventually lose their confidence.

How can I possibly choose a dish in this restaurant when there are over two hundred entrées to choose from?

Never before have we had so many options and so much information to help guide us in the process of selecting which options to pursue. We have had an explosion of information that in theory should help us all make better decisions, including how to take care of ourselves more effectively. Unfortunately, as anyone who has attempted to research a problem on the Internet knows quite well, having millions of resources and opinions on a matter can lead to more confusion and ultimately more anxiety, rather than simplifying our quest for clarity and confidence in our choices. This is not a new state of affairs, which we can recognize when we return to the work of our patron, Dr. Freud. He pointed out that our thought processes are governed by certain general principles, and he was highly successful in understanding his patients' behavior. His insights, however, relied on a treatment program that most of us would shy away from in modern day society.

So, Herr Doktor Freud, what is it that really makes people tick?

The practice of psychoanalysis, which entailed five hours of individual sessions each week and would last for many years, is predicated on the idea that everyone has a built-in set of variables, some conscious and many submerged, which determine how we deal with any given situation. Because many of our desires and motivations are unconscious, there is generally no simple cause-and-effect relationship between our conscious, stated desires and our actions. So, as Freud pointed out, to many scientists' great dismay, we are not nearly as much in control of our thoughts and behaviors as was once hoped in the age of enlightenment.

The model that Freud proposed does not conform to the medical model, in which a fairly clear-cut trigger leads to a specific outcome. A patient is exposed to strep bacteria and ends up with strep throat. Another patient eats too much fatty food, which leads to gallstones and subsequently to surgery to remove the gallbladder. Of course it's not usually that simple in the world of healthcare, but the medical model requires that we select a single primary cause for the patient's condition.

Why do I say those terrible things when I get angry with my boyfriend (or girlfriend)?

To add insult to injury, our unconscious motivations are not the only impediment to rational behavior. The other major obstacle we face is our own emotional state. The more anxiety or stress we encounter in any given situation, the more these mysterious unconscious factors come into play. If you were to ask someone in advance, on a hypothetical basis, how they would handle a given issue, my guess is that their response in the imaginary scenario would likely be rational, well thought out, and even a bit heroic at times. In other words, their imagined or fantasized response will often differ from their real-life response. While we all tend to view ourselves as being cool under pressure, this is not always so easy. Here is a striking and tragic example of this phenomenon:

> A bright, twenty-seven-year-old woman who had a history of panic attacks was at home sleeping when her kitchen caught on fire. Once she woke up and smelled smoke, she found her roommate, who was calling for her to join her in another upstairs bedroom. The roommate urged her to wait for help to arrive. . Rather than staying in this safe location for rescuers, however, she became panicked and attempted to leave the house in the peak of the fire. Overcome by flames and smoke, she lost consciousness and suffered extensive third-degree burns. Her roommate was unable to retrieve her due to the flames, and ultimately exited the home by ladder, assisted by a firefighter. She was treated preemptively for smoke inhalation, with no long-term harm from the fire.

Now, most of us would vehemently claim to be in the roommate's camp, meaning that we would clearly make the right decision in this sad circumstance. In many cases, however, anxiety arouses the primitive irrational parts of the brain, which often leads to a fight-or-flight response. This level of the brain, which we essentially share with reptiles, birds, and other much less developed animals, does not recognize logic or reason. Only self-preservation and survival enter into the equation in these scenarios.

> When I rescued that child in the burning house, it was almost like a dream. I didn't even think about what I was doing.

In this case you would probably recognize that many decisions, which would come easily in the context of a calm and relaxed discussion, become more erratic in the moment of truth. Many individuals who appear quite average and unassuming rise to the occasion and act in a heroic fashion. Others who appear seasoned and resourceful seem to struggle in the face of adversity. This pattern of course explains the rationale for rehearsing at great length for any emotionally charged or potentially overwhelming situation. Those of us who have participated in dozens of fire drills or who have established emergency plans for our homes are more likely to follow our plan, rather than relying on primitive responses that might lead us into more danger. So we would generally accept that too much emotional arousal can disrupt our ability to focus on making a sound decision, just as too much static or feedback in a microphone can limit our ability to hear what the speaker is saying.

The power of the unconscious, or, "But officer, I swear I was only doing 55, not 80!"

In psychiatry, it is understood that each decision that we make, or fail to make, is influenced by a multitude of conflicting inputs. So, ultimately I enjoy taking on the challenging and often quixotic task of attempting to analyze—and, I hope, coming to understand—my patients' motivations and impulses, many of which lead to complications, which in turn lead them to my office in search of help and insight. As examples, here are some statements that I have heard repeatedly over the years, many of which may be familiar to the average reader:

> "I don't even know what that argument [actually a major blowout with his wife the day before] was about."

> "Something snapped, and I just lost it."

> "I don't know what the devil made me tell my wife that she's gained weight. It was crazy."

> "I live for going fishing—though I can't tell you how many years it's been since I went."

"I know I wrote that suicide note, but I promise—I didn't mean a word of it. I was just mad that my husband came home at 10:00 p.m. again."

"I can't believe I got fired!" (A statement from a patient who had been miserable in his job for several years and was planning to quit "any day now.")

"I didn't plan to have anything to drink last night, but somehow things just got away from me." (Words spoken by a patient who was arrested for driving under the influence after having at least twelve drinks at a wedding.)

"I really meant to use that money for a new car." (Words of regret from a young patient who had spent over $25,000 gambling on various sports events.)

In summary these comments reflect how little control we have over our behavior at times. And, while it takes most of us quite some time to save up $25,000 or to land a desirable job, it takes only one or two poor decisions to fritter away large sums or to lose the boss's favor. Like a storm that washes away decades of accumulated sand, a short period of indiscretion can lead to major financial, vocational, marital, or legal setbacks.

Are mentally ill people really a different sort of species?

This misconception seems to be rooted in the public's discomfort with the concept of mental illness. Somehow anxiety and mood disorders have become modern-day forms of leprosy, to be ostracized and avoided at all costs. The commonly observed practice of telling others that one is "fine" in a superficial manner is likely another result of this discomfort. This reluctance to accept that psychiatric disorders can in fact affect anyone remains widespread, presenting a major obstacle to the public's understanding and acceptance of our field. We often overhear an argument that may have become heated leading to dismissive or demeaning statements such as, "You're just crazy." Or, "I bet you didn't take your medication today." This is one surefire way of squelching almost any meaningful interaction.

So clearly we as a society tend to use the concept of mental illness as a means of demonstrating our normalcy or superiority in a typically judgmental manner. But the fact is that we are all affected with the same conditions, feelings, and experiences—it's just a matter of degree. The patients whom I evaluate and treat are generally dealing with more severe versions of everyday challenges that we all face. The following chart illustrates this point:

Normal Variant	Mental disorder
Getting the blues	Severe depressive disorder
Being a perfectionist	Obsessive compulsive personality disorder
Being moody	Bipolar disorder
Having trust issues	Paranoid psychosis
Worrying about your health	Being a hypochondriac
Checking to make sure you turned off the range once	Checking the range fifty-two times and getting to work two hours late (Obsessive compulsive disorder)

From these common examples you can see that the problems I address in my practice tend to present on a continuum, meaning that they vary enormously in severity. Thus a mild symptom (left column above), which most of us would consider normal, can escalate to the point that the individual is either in distress, is unable to function well, or is inflicting distress on those around him or her (right column). We could then declare that we have entered the realm of mental illness.

But it would never happen to me!

While most of us can accept (though, in general, not comfortably) that we might someday end up with appendicitis or pneumonia or some similar medical condition, we somehow tend to feel immune to emotional disorders. Over the years, many of my patients have expressed feelings of disbelief or even shock when they were informed of their diagnosis:

> "I've never been a depressed person. Suddenly I could barely get out of bed. I was sure it was some sort of hormonal thing. Or maybe Lyme disease."

"I was doing so well last year. I had a great job, a great house, a great wife, and great kids. I had just got a nice raise and a promotion. So when I went on that drinking binge, I turned into somebody totally different. It wasn't me."

"I used to travel around the world with just a backpack and a few dollars. I didn't even worry about things that might happen to me. Now I can't even leave the house without having to take a bunch of medication. And even then I'm still scared stiff."

These patients did not expect to develop mood or anxiety disorders. They were just like you and me—except for their vulnerability to psychiatric conditions when placed under enough pressure, at the appropriate age of onset. Often I am concerned that the person becomes defined or limited by these disorders rather than viewing the disease process as a challenge that can be managed or even brought into full remission. Many patients comment that they are no longer "the same person" they were prior to their diagnosis. In this case I attempt to modify their thinking so they can react in the same way that they might to any physical or other setback.

An important point here is that, in the short term, treatment for a specific disorder often fails to return the patient to his/her full level of functional ability. It is thus critical that a patient be aware of— and receive—full rehabilitative services to help address any residual deficits that might have arisen during an episode of illness. In fact, most patients who are treated for an acute episode of psychosis, depression, or mania will require three to six months to recuperate fully. Without effective treatment and education it may take much longer, to the point that the patient is likely to suffer serious setbacks in his/her work, relationships, and finances that might have been prevented if he or she'd had adequate access to services. Though many of my patients hope to put their difficulties behind them and are confident that they will not relapse, we know that any individual with a given condition is likely to relapse, given enough time, stress, and biological vulnerability. We also know that, with many medical conditions, such as strokes, heart attacks, pneumonia, etc., it takes considerable time after short-term stabilization for the patient to feel that he or she is back to 100 percent, physically and emotionally. In the case of a patient who is actively seeking out support and other resources, recovery moves much more quickly, and relapse is much less likely.

Why can't I just take some Xanax whenever I have a bad day and just deal with things like everyone else?

The concept of being "stressed out' is of course common parlance, with a trend for our impatient and at times unrealistic society to expect immediate relief of any distress. We are trained by the media and by marketing campaigns to expect prompt solutions for our ills, whether, medical, financial, emotional or spiritual. It thus becomes tempting to simply avail ourselves of a short-term treatment (thought often short-lived) rather than viewing ourselves as potentially mentally ill. The fact is that many remedies work quite rapidly and thus lead the patient to view their discomfort as a short-term concern, rather than a meaningful and persistent condition which merits diagnosis and ongoing therapy.

So what if my son's a little weird? He's just different—there's nothing wrong with him!

Naturally we appreciate that everyone has a right to their idiosyncrasies and foibles, especially those of us with power, wealth, or other forms of influence. Even kings and presidents, however, can be labeled mentally ill. In fact, some forms of mood disorders seem helpful in this regard. Consider how many celebrities, authors, artists, or politicians have been thought to have suffered from bipolar disorder (formerly known as manic depression)? Just think how much could be accomplished by a bright individual with boundless energy, no need for sleep or meals, a speeding intellect, and minimal or no patience for anyone who stands in their way? This would enable one to conquer the world—if only it didn't come to an end. Unfortunately, the energy of the manic individual is at times misdirected and instead takes the form of anger, paranoia, or severe grandiosity. Occasionally I have had the rare pleasure of evaluating patients who presented with the more classical form of mania. These high-powered individuals often describe—with much excitement—thousands of brilliant schemes coursing through their minds and enjoy an intense feeling of euphoria. (Just think of the best day of your life and multiply by a hundred.)

Why does everyone in movies, politics, or the six o'clock news seem to be bipolar?

If you consider the usual tabloid headline, movie plot, or even cocktail party conversation, you might wonder at the number of references to some sort of psychiatric disorder. Somehow, as a society, we find this topic fascinating. Of course the media is highly gifted at providing us with what sells. And, since we generally find others' seemingly irrational behavior rewarding to read about, marvel at with our friends, and analyze as lay psychoanalysts, behavioral disturbances frequently pop up in in these arenas. If no one suffered from mental illness, and everyone always had a level mood, along with entirely predictable and logical behavior, readership of our papers and magazines would surely decline precipitously. What a monotonous and tedious world that would be! This does not mean that I endorse efforts to avoid treating psychiatric disorders, but rather that much of what makes our society diverse and meaningful might result from actions and decisions that are based on some variant of a psychiatric condition. But of course you might argue that I am biased, having chosen to practice in this field.

What's wrong with being a little unstable? It's no fun to be normal!

This is an intriguing argument, one that I have heard countless times in my prior role as an inpatient psychiatrist. As the primary arbiter of who remains in the hospital and who is released in the course of the day (assisted, of course, by the entire treatment team, comprised of nurses, social workers, recreation therapists, psychologists, and the unit chief, who all have input into this assessment process), I have entertained hundreds of accounts, explanations, and rationalizations for a wide variety of dangerous, uncharacteristic, and impulsive behavior. Patients who are fearful of being labeled as mentally ill, who worry that they will face weeks in a locked unit, or who simply don't believe that there is any real solution for their problems tend to find many creative ways of explaining their actions. If they do ultimately admit to the decisions that led to their admission to the hospital, they generally identify many triggers that they claim would have led anyone to react in a similar fashion. It is only when we include family members, friends, coworkers, or neighbors in this process that the real story emerges. Clearly, we often minimize our irrational behavior as a response to related embarrassment, shame, or stigma. Fortunately we have seen some progress in this area, with many prominent authors, actors, politicians, physicians, and other dignitaries going public with their mental illnesses.

But why does it seem that everyone on TV or in the movies is taking Prozac and/or seeing a therapist?

I have always been struck by the general public's fascination with my field of choice. Much of our modern media, whether in films, newspapers, novels, tabloids, etc. seems to focus on human behavior—or, for the most part, misbehavior. How many movies or books can you recall that fail to include at least one character who appears to be manic, psychotic, morbidly depressed, or panic-stricken? Whenever the plot seems to be struggling to find a new twist to keep the audience on the edge of its seat, a previously unremarkable character has decided to stop taking his lithium. So then it's off to the races, with a manic but photogenic and well-groomed character who is in hot pursuit of his best friend's wife.

Yet in these depictions there often appears to be a lack of understanding about psychiatric issues. Most well-meaning patients, families, or friends toss around terms in a confident manner yet when pressed are not able to explain their meaning. A neighbor speaks of his boss being "bipolar." Another friend tells me of her "panic attacks" when her daughter is serving in a volleyball match. A colleague refers to his partner's "bad case of OCD," which somehow keeps him from finishing his work efficiently. A patient speaks of her mother-in-law as "totally psychotic." A neighbor speaks of his wife's "nervous breakdown." Yet these terms are quite different in a clinical setting than in their everyday colloquial usage.

When asked about these concepts, most people appear confident about their command of these terms and seem perplexed or even annoyed when I present a different point of view. Even though there are many resources and diagnostic manuals that promise to clarify and standardize our understanding of mental disease, many studies have demonstrated that when ten expert psychiatrists are asked for a diagnosis, they are far from unanimous. With certain disorders, fewer than half the specialists from any given group were in agreement. We assume, erroneously, that everyone—physicians, patients, and their advocates—will all wind up on the same page.

As a side note, we also tend to accept the media's portrayal of mental illness as gospel. If we see it on TV or on the Internet, it must be true. To demonstrate this principle, I would like to relate an event that occurred several years ago at the annual conference of the American Psychiatric Association. The actress Lorraine Bracco, who artfully portrayed Tony Soprano's psychiatrist, was a guest speaker at this event, and she presented her perspective on her work in the HBO series. In an intriguing twist, the highly educated specialists who attended this event posed many complex questions regarding psychoanalytic theories in the question-and-answer part of her presentation. They seemingly forgot that she was simply a gifted actress who was playing the part of a psychoanalyst and began to view her as an expert psychiatric colleague. This supports my point that the American public tends to blindly accept whatever it reads or hears in the media. Our citizens have largely lost track of the old dictum that you can't believe everything that you read (or see on TV, the Internet, or your Twitter account).

For this loss of our critical faculties and excessive credulity we could blame several culprits. In the media many self-pronounced experts bandy about psychiatric terms, with little meaningful discussion of their exact meaning. Being 100 percent truthful, could you actually define the commonplace term "codependent?" I would propose that ten individuals would come up with ten different explanations. And even our so-called experts would likely disagree on many aspects of these commonly used terms. Then, of course, we all (at least those of us who are honest) can relate to some extent to many of these disorders, having either recognized some features in ourselves, in our friends, or more commonly, in our adversaries. For example, when we choose an accountant to track our income and minimize our tax burden, we would clearly favor one who is meticulous to the point that he or she pores over our 1040 to ferret out any possible deductions. Does that mean that our CPA has an obsessive compulsive personality? Possibly, but in this case this form of adaptation would work in our favor. When we choose a surgeon to perform a kidney transplant, we would tend to be more comfortable with a physician who is self-promoting and confident to the point that we might label him or her as narcissistic. We would tend to shy away from an overly modest and self-effacing specialist who fails to inspire us with his or her ability to perform an intrinsically challenging and dangerous procedure.

So you are implying that mental illness can be viewed in a positive light?

This line of reasoning simply reinforces the idea, initially presented by Freud, that any symptom or adaptation serves a purpose, though this might initially be difficult to surmise. Those of us who find rewards in poring over financial statements and spreadsheets might find an obsessive compulsive adaptation helpful. However, the CPA who requires three weeks to review and submit a simple 1040 (if such a thing exists) might find him- or herself on the unemployment line around March or April. So, in our initial understanding of mental illness, the individual must have either substantial distress or significant functional deficits, or often both. In either case, the condition becomes a liability. In many cases, we find that the patient fails to view himself as suffering from a disorder but is viewed by others as dysfunctional.

What about stigma and ostracism—as in One Flew over the Cuckoo's Nest?

When we want to discredit or diminish another person without actually presenting valid arguments or logic, we often resort to casting doubt on that person's mental health. This tactic was perfected in the Soviet Union, as well as in Washington, DC, where many dissidents were labeled as schizophrenic. In many past political campaigns, opposing candidates were often smeared as somehow defective or untrustworthy because of a fully resolved past episode of depression or even any prior form of psychiatric treatment. Finally, the fact remains that the study of human behavior is quite complex and poorly understood, with limited objective progress since the writings of the father of psychiatry, Sigmund Freud. Even though we speak of "chemical imbalances" as well as serotonin and other biological factors, any honest and humble student of this field would acknowledge that we have actually mastered perhaps ten percent of what there is to know about the workings of the human mind. Just the idea that the sum total of human knowledge, emotions, and dreams could be generated by a small, wrinkled organ is in fact mind-boggling.

Chapter 2

The Art of Psychiatric Diagnosis, or "How bad is it, Doc? Am I losing my mind?"

How do I determine my psychiatric diagnosis, or whether I even have one?

We have a simple means of breaking down disorders in our field. While there are some rare categories such as perversions, the vast majority of everyday conditions are included in the following broad categories::

- Mood disorders
- Anxiety disorders
- Psychotic disorders
- Impulse control disorders
- Addiction disorders

These terms are all widely used and fairly self-explanatory, although in the real world we often encounter confusion. This can result from the fact that many conditions can fall into more than one category. The next point is that many patients have more than one clinical disorder, which we refer to as co-morbidity. Lastly, in order to arrive at a confident diagnosis, two conditions must be met:

1) The patient has to be medically cleared, meaning that s/he is not suffering from an underlying medical or surgical disorder that would account for his/her symptoms.

2) His/her behavior does not result from a state of intoxication with any substance.

Subsequent chapters will outline in some detail each class of disorders, though of course in the real world there tends to be much overlap between these areas. Thus, most patients with mood disorders also have some diagnosable anxiety disorder. Most patients with addiction issues also struggle with impulse control. People who are incapable of managing their impulses usually find that life becomes much more complicated. Given enough time and opportunity, then, they generally tend to develop substantial anxiety.

The other rule is that we cannot label any given individual with a disorder based on our own emotional reactions or judgment. So the neighbor who refers to his boss as "bipolar" cannot confidently state his case without clear-cut evidence (though most of us take pleasure in diagnosing anyone who raises our blood pressure). In this case, then, the process would require establishing that the aforementioned boss is either consistently unhappy or that he has considerable difficulty performing his duties for extended periods as a result of his specific disorder. In summary, it is critical to note that patients must either be suffering distress as a result of their illness or have substantial difficulty functioning, or most commonly both. The fact that we have an eccentric neighbor or that our uncle loses his temper three times a day does not suffice to prove that they are psychiatrically impaired. From a practical point of view, the functional impairment can be academic, social, or vocational and is generally obvious to the individual's family, boss or peers.

When does behavior go from being odd to being pathological?

The key principle here is that these disorders exist on a continuum, from mild or subclinical to severe. Most, if not all, of us can identify mood swings from time to time—if not in ourselves, then in the people around us. We've also had days in which we did not function at our usual level. So when does the problem become a clinical disorder? This is where our field can become a bit murky. To the credit of my selfless academic peers, there are many scales and assessments that can help sort this out. It turns out that we can measure distress in many different ways. So if I tell you that I had a bad day, the experts could actually place a number on it. If a patient tends to stick his head in the sand, telling me he never has a bad day, the next step is to inquire if he has been fully enjoying his social and recreational activities. If an avid fishing enthusiast has not been out on the water for six months, then I would contend that he is not at his usual level of happiness. A doting grandmother who has not wanted to see her grandchildren over the past month is likely to meet the criteria for a mood disorder.

On the other hand, many of us are either too busy to focus on our own state of well-being, are self-sacrificing types who focus on the welfare of others, or just are not accustomed to the luxury of doing a self-assessment. We may face pressure to the point that we are not able to experience feelings but rather must conserve our mental energy just to get by. Some psychologists have described this as a form of being on autopilot that seems to enable us to function even under duress. You might view this as analogous to the state of shock that often accompanies severe physical trauma. This is what we refer to as "isolation of affect," a state in which we are unaware of our feelings. If we enter our office in a sad or nervous mood, the task is to maintain a facade so that our coworkers or supervisor are tricked into thinking that we are just peachy, thank you very much. So in that case, the often reluctant patient will state categorically that he rarely experiences any feelings of sadness or distress, and if he does, these feelings are fleeting.

> "I was doing fine, going to work, bringing home my paycheck, playing with the kids. Then, when I was downsized, everything fell apart. I worked so many years for that company, and they had the nerve to just offer me a severance check and tell me to clean out my desk. I can't stop thinking about it. Sometimes I find myself thinking about ending it all."

course most sixteen-year-olds do appear to be possessed by some sort of extraterrestrial being). By the same token, those of you who have steered clear of substance abuse issues by that stage of development are usually on fairly solid ground.

Does that mean it's all downhill once I make it into my thirties?

Unfortunately I cannot make the same claims for either mood or anxiety disorders, which will afflict many, if not most, of us in our middle or late years. For example, we've all joked about the inevitable midlife crisis, which is a rite of passage for most of us, to varying degrees. And of course it is not surprising that an elderly individual who may be facing retirement, chronic medical illness, loss of a spouse, or a sense of being overlooked by society might face a considerable risk of developing a depressive episode. Please see the section on special populations in the chapter on obstacles to treatment, which will discuss treatment concerns of the elderly in more detail.

Chapter 3

When to Seek Treatment, or "Why should I bother dealing with my problems? No one else does!"

Sadly, this chapter is aptly titled. It has been estimated and confirmed in many studies that, at most, only a third of patients with significant—and diagnosable— mental health conditions actually seek out treatment. Even more striking, of those who do, only about a third are ultimately treated effectively. So this is a real obstacle that surfaces in my practice virtually every day. Between any given individual's reluctance to accept that he may need—or at least benefit from—my services and the vagaries of our health care system, it is remarkable (at least to my unjaded eyes) when a new patient actually arrives at my office and requests a thorough evaluation. Often it is necessary for a disorder to attain crisis proportions to catalyze this process. Often my assistant finds herself bombarded with a variety of anxious—and at times demanding—callers, who have finally decided to take action ... pronto. "Can you see my husband today?" "Do you take my insurance? Why not? I have really good insurance." "Will my boss find out I'm seeing a psychiatrist?" "Will the medication turn me into a zombie?" "Will I end up losing my job, or will they cancel my health insurance policy?"

I guess I should have come in twenty years ago.

The concerns are all real obstacles in the world of health care, many of which derive from entrenched preconceptions and the stigma related to mental illness. These attitudes often limit our ability to admit that we might be suffering from a mental health disorder. So from this you might surmise that the majority of my patients wait until they reach a crisis, just like the fearful patient who waits until he develops an abscess before consulting a dentist. Or the obese smoker who fails to take action until he develops crushing chest pain. Many reluctant patients are compelled to find my office due to an ultimatum from their immediate family, supervisor, or some other authority figure. It just so happens that this figure is usually a woman. For some reason, even in the advanced age of the Internet and our greater biological understanding of mood, anxiety, and addiction disorders, men somehow remain opposed to acknowledging emotional issues and taking action. Is this a form of denial or some strain of machismo or some legacy of the Wild West? Or could it simply be a lack of awareness that these conditions do exist and can be addressed in a rational and effective fashion?

Why does it seem as if everyone and his dog are taking Prozac?

I like to think that the increased use of antianxiety and antidepressant agents is based on three factors:

1) Reduced stigma and increased support of those who seek out treatment

2) Increased availability due to expanded insurance coverage

3) Increased awareness and education in our communities and institutions

Of course, a more skeptical analysis might point to three less positive trends:

1) A barrage of advertising and direct consumer marketing that is persuading even those of us who suffer from subclinical forms of these conditions to move forward with treatment

2) A higher level of overall stress and frustration in modern-day society

3) An unwillingness to work through issues, with a preference for simply medicating them away, just as many disgruntled employees might mix a martini at the end of the day rather than determining whether it's time to find a new position or have a talk with the boss.

What about the "stiff upper lip" approach?

I would argue that all of these factors come into play. We all have the option of postponing any response to problems until they reach crisis proportions. I often regretfully inform my patients that I do not expect them to modify their behavior or attitudes based on good intentions alone. One has to experience considerable discomfort or frustration in order to question and modify longstanding patterns of behavior. In general we tend to come up with a game plan and stick with it—at least until we realize that we are losing the game by a large margin.

"I'm not too happy with my job, but it pays the bills. The lawyers I work for treat me like dirt. I'd like to find a better office situation, but I hear the job market is pretty poor. I hope I'll find something in the next few months."

Once we find ourselves in severe distress, and we can no longer present a confident facade to the world, then change and growth are finally possible. In real life we refer to this phenomenon as having to reach crisis proportions, or what the addiction community refers to as "hitting rock bottom." Then of course all bets are off, and we enter survival mode. Whatever it takes to "get you through the night" becomes acceptable and logical. Many of us rely on various short-term fixes, such as self-medicating with alcohol or drugs. Others will engage in other self-destructive behavior, such as smoking too much, driving too fast, or yelling at the family dog. Still others will start to question their relationships, their jobs, their homes, and their families, in search of what could be making them feel so anxious or distressed. Many of us will just tough it out. We keep on waking up, going to work, paying our bills, and doing whatever is necessary to get by. But this is not the goal—to live a life of "quiet desperation." Or to turn on some sort of autopilot mode, which protects us from having to think too much or feel too much. So the failure to take on a psychiatric disorder can be quite costly. Not in the sense that most patients end up going bankrupt or losing their homes, even though some do. Most don't end up losing their families or jobs, though some do. From my perspective, the saddest commentary has come from many of my patients, who look back on their depressions from a new perspective. When they are fully recovered, they look back on the time when they suffered the most, and often tell me, "I wish I had found some kind of treatment years ago."

These disorders are capable of robbing time, the most precious commodity. They can take the pleasure from our everyday activities and interactions. They can limit our ability to focus on our work or personal goals. They can lead us to seek a divorce in spite of a generally healthy relationship, or to leave a reasonably fulfilling job, based on our sense of dissatisfaction and ennui. In a more serious and insidious manner, they can steal our sense of confidence, of hope, of who we are, and what we have to offer the world.

Why can't these patients just snap out of it?

Many patients who fail to seek help feel unworthy of being helped. They often believe that their mood disorder is some form of punishment meted out from above due to some long-past sin that they might have committed. As thinking creatures, we often attempt to explain how the world operates. If we become ill with no clear trigger for this, we struggle to find a reason. If someone develops a functional or mood disorder, then we might ask ourselves whether that person is lazy or burned out or just doesn't want to work. It is difficult to make sense of a person who isolates him- or herself, who remains in bed, who doesn't seem to want to help him- or herself. We know that it would be important for that person to take action, so why doesn't he or she? Only after interviewing thousands of depressed and hopeless patients have I come to understand their sense of helplessness, of being stuck, of weighing a thousand pounds, of feeling that the outside world will only beat them down even further. So this starts to make more sense.

These disorders change one's behavior, clearly, but they act primarily by modifying one's way of thinking. For someone who feels that his or her illness is terminal, that there is no effective cure, it would be logical to retreat, just as a cat who is ill will withdraw from his family until he either mends or succumbs to his condition.

Most of my patients are fearful of posing a burden to their loved ones. They worry that their declining mood will prove contagious or that others will label them as "lazy," "weak," or somehow unmotivated. They are aware that their loved ones are concerned, frustrated, or even exasperated with their lack of improvement. Many of them have had mixed experiences in their past treatments, with disconcerting accounts of therapists or psychiatrists who offered little hope and even less guidance. They have often made efforts to locate treatment centers but might encounter significant obstacles in this process. When they arrive at my office, I find it helpful to acknowledge their frustration. In addition, I often point out that the field of psychiatry is imperfect, with inconsistent results and only partially effective medications and schools of psychotherapy. Ultimately I emphasize, however, that virtually all patients can expect positive results within a reasonable period of time, given adequate time and commitment.

Although we know that many cases of anxiety or depression will subside with time and support, those who lack support or who make decisions that have a negative impact on their lives face a treacherous process. For this reason I am grateful for the publicity and advertising that the pharmaceutical companies support in the media. Even though I am aware that this is designed to help them gain more market share and is not entirely altruistic, I remain indebted to them for educating patients about these conditions and about the fact that we do have effective treatments.

Why do I get stuck on the sofa so often?

This is an excellent question that reflects the central conundrum of mental illness. Those of us who are suffering from medical conditions tend to benefit, for the most part, from withdrawing. Anyone who suggested that I could have gone to the office when I had the flu would be profoundly misguided. When a patient has fevers, shaking, anorexia, nausea, and vomiting, few bosses—even tyrannical ones—would expect them to show up at work. Those patients who are suffering emotionally often fail to elicit much sympathy, however. To my patients with severe panic attacks, hopelessness, racing thoughts, and flights of ideas, it is logical to take a leave of absence. Clearly they would not be successful in the office setting and are better off making themselves scarce. Their lack of focus, limited confidence, and fatigue—common symptoms that tend to accompany most cases of mood disorder—would surely raise the ire of even reasonable supervisors. For this reason, most of my patients are sorely tempted to call in sick. They make excuses when invited to social events. At times they even pass up opportunities to spend time with their closest friends or even their grandchildren. In the long run, however, this pattern of withdrawal can actually feed a mood disorder. A given individual who isolates and therefore lacks social or recreational stimulation has a considerable risk of developing a chronic mood disorder.

On the other hand, that person might be difficult to convince that his or her condition will improve in the outside world. Many of them fear losing their jobs, families, or other critical supports and resources. For this reason we make every effort, in both inpatient and outpatient settings, to engage our patients as much as possible. Our nurses and recreation therapists tirelessly exhort them to leave the comfort of their bed or the sofa. We work incessantly to interest them in regular interactions, meals, sleep, and exercise. In the early phases of treatment we often feel guilty for pushing a patient who clearly feels overwhelmed and incapable of mustering the energy to socialize with or meet new peers. But in my experience, the vast majority of patients come to appreciate our exhortations several days later, when their energy level is higher and they are once again able to enjoy the support of peers and family members. Those patients who resist our efforts and continue to isolate have a diminished range of options. Should they fail to maintain a basic level of family support, they often become isolated and assume a high risk of chronic illness.

Worrying - Ameica's least-favorite pastime

You might ask the obvious question based on the above section. If my patients are in bed most of the day and night, how do they occupy their time? Over the past two decades, I haven't found many of them reading Russian novels or doing oil painting. They aren't learning a new language or designing the next Facebook. What I tend to find in most cases is that they are caught up in a strangely addictive behavior— constant worrying. Though on the surface this doesn't appear very gratifying, it is an extremely common response to stress. If we have a pile of paperwork to process before tax day—and today happens to be April 2)—we often find ourselves procrastinating. How do we attack that pile of financial statements in the study? Where do we even begin?

What, me worry? You bet your petooties!

> "I'm so embarrassed about the situation. I'm actually a bookkeeper, and I know all about this stuff. But when I started working part-time, they paid me pretty well. I was putting away maybe fifty bucks a week."

This leads to a state of feeling overwhelmed, which in turn can lead to paralysis. So instead of taking action, we start to dwell on the difficulty or unpleasant nature of the task before us. Then, when we run out of steam worrying about tax day, we find other areas of concern. Did our teenage son get his homework done? Did we ever change the oil in the family vehicle? Did we forget to pay the Visa bill? On and on, until we have spent the day worrying and accomplished nothing. Then naturally we look back and worry about how the day floated by with no significant progress with our goals or objectives. What if this happens again tomorrow? And the day after that? Ultimately we will end up in a lot of trouble, which easily becomes a vicious cycle, since, soon enough, we have valid reasons to worry. I have patients who have failed to file income tax returns for nine or more years yet are embarrassed to consult an accountant, request assistance from the IRS, or enlist their families or friends in an effort to catch up. Even if an amnesty program presents itself, they fail to take action.

Others have gradually arrived at a point at which they lose focus on their own needs and wishes. They fail to engage in their favorite pastimes and neglect to set up social events. Of course, as long as they are going to work, paying the bills, and just keeping the house running at a reasonable level, they can often tolerate this trend for months or even years. Ultimately, however, there is a cost in lost recreation, limited support, and missed opportunities. This can lead to burnout, which again can be tolerated for some time. Alternatively, the individual might present to his or her primary care doctor with a stress-induced disorder such as high blood pressure. Still others might complain to their spouse or possibly their doctor about more vague concerns. They just don't sleep well at night. They have disturbing dreams. Perhaps their energy is low, and they spend the day in bed on Sundays. Their libido is missing, and their partner is questioning whether they have a medical issue or might be losing interest in the relationship. These are all reflections of the simple fact that we tend to do what we have to do but fail to recognize that taking care of ourselves should ideally be our top priority. If I raise these concerns, the patient might feel even more pressure to make time for recreation, come up with funds to pay for outings, etc. This unfortunately might place him or her under even more pressure, which can retrigger the cycle of worrying.

Plus, the fact remains that life is complicated. The level of stress out there has never been higher, in spite of the medical, technological and political progress we have made over the past hundred years. Who can possibly keep up with everything these days? We have more information to digest, more bills to pay, more doomsayers who warn us of impending climate change, financial meltdowns, negative societal changes, and political gridlock and corruption. For many of these and other reasons, the act of worrying is universally recognized as a reasonably valid use of our time. For the most part, people realize the incorrectness of simply telling someone to relax, and not to worry any more. Plus, worrying itself is not an easy pastime. Those of us who worry much of the time tend to feel fatigued and depleted at the end of the day, even if they haven't taken action or checked off any goals on their to-do list. Worrying is quite draining, even if it doesn't require getting out of the easy chair.

What happens to worrywarts?

As I noted above, those who engage in chronic worrying tend to be less productive, since much of their time and energy is channeled into the process of managing a stream of negative thoughts and fears. Plus chronic untreated anxiety often leads to a variety of responses or "coping skills." Most worriers indulge in a range of classic behaviors --some potentially self-destructive and others fairly benign. At times patients are able to rise to the occasion and come up with appropriate and adaptive behaviors, such as exercise, social events, spiritual commitments or even a well-deserved siesta. On the other hand, many of us are not so wise in our choices. We end up resorting to a variety of unhealthy activities, which the individual hopes – often in vain - will relieve his or her anxiety. You might view these behaviors as reasonable means of coping, though these are not often successful solutions for managing stress. I classify these behaviors in three categories:

1) **Self-medicating,** which might include the use of alcohol, drugs such as caffeine, or cigarettes.
2) **Distractions,** such as setting up excessive commitments, making extensive lists, shopping, or spending extra time at the office.
3) **Avoidance**, such as isolating, remaining in bed, watching excessive TV, using Internet etc. Other common behaviors could include changing jobs or relationships with no clear rationale

Of course these behaviors all share a common feature: they allow us to avoid taking the bull by the horns. Rather than dealing with an imposing issue head-on, we instead sidestep it and put it off for some undetermined period of time. You could call this escapism or avoidance or procrastination. The fact is that we are all guilty of these behaviors at times, since we cannot possibly do it all in one day. So at the end of the day the main concern is that we have left many critical or essential tasks undone, to the point that our level of worrying—and related avoidance behavior—flares up even more the following day. When we speak of healthy means of reducing pressure, such as heading down to the Bahamas, going to a Lakers game, or spending an afternoon in the spa, we usually have to be prepared to bring a large sum of money and to make use of our precious paid leave in order to access this enviable but costly mode of stress management.

I have at times worked with well-meaning individuals who keep detailed lists of important goals or activities. On the surface we would find this effort commendable, with no cause for criticism. But unfortunately, this activity can become a form of worrying, which at times serves to delay action by channeling one's energy into the endless formulation and compilation of more and more lists.

Can stress really kill me?

This is a common (usually unspoken) concern, which of course could be considered an "old wives' tale" such as the idea that you can catch the flu because you forgot your galoshes and got your feet wet. This, however, has in fact been a perennial—if often implicit fear—of our culture as a whole. "You'd better relax, or you'll have a heart attack!" (That's a really helpful comment, however well-intentioned.) "Just get ahold of yourself!" "Your blood pressure's gonna hit the roof if you don't take a chill pill!" We all want to be stress-free, and there is actually a scientific basis for fearing stress itself. Those of us who are constantly in an aroused or hypervigilant state, with our fight-or-flight response activated, are in fact at risk for a variety of medical and emotional setbacks. As the body girds for battle, there are several immediate and dramatic responses. First, our adrenal glands start pumping away, releasing potent hormones that raise our heart rate and our level of alertness. Next, the body steers all resources away from nonessential functions, such as eating, eliminating waste, etc. Finally, the body is equipped with more resources to help make a getaway—more oxygen arrives at the muscles, a higher respiratory rate helps clear carbon dioxide, and the liver helps break down energy stores.

Physiological responses to stress

- Release of epinephrine and norepinephrine from adrenal glands

- Release of cortisol from pituitary gland, leading to increased availability of glucose to fuel muscles and brain

- Elevation of heart rate and blood pressure, leading to increased blood flow to muscles and brain. This results from response number 1.

- Suppression of appetite and sexual behavior

In the short term, this state of arousal, which we often label as fight or flight, is usually well tolerated and does not appear to compromise an individual's longevity, apart from those unfortunate individuals who suffer heart attacks when facing a very frightening or physically demanding event. In the long term, however, a high level of stress hormones has been proven to accelerate damage to the lining of our arteries, thus increasing the risk of a stroke or heart attack. There is also growing support for the theory that stress will trigger the secretion of copious levels of steroids, mainly cortisol, which can predispose a given individual to diabetes, osteoporosis, weight gain, a weakened immune system, and other conditions. The answer to the above question is thus a qualified "yes," in that we will likely face premature illness or possibly even death if we neglect our elevated stress levels. From this standpoint, what my colleagues and I practice is a form of preventive care, since so many medical disorders are triggered or exacerbated by stress. These have in fact been well documented for over ninety years as the aptly named psychosomatic disorders.

What about if I never get stressed out?

Many of my patients, and I myself, have to admit to being envious of those West Coast surfer types who never seem to break a sweat. Are there actually real people out there who never have a bad day or who never lose sleep in spite of everyday pressures, hassles, and concerns? Many well-organized studies have noted that most of us have a certain set point for happiness or anxiety. Many individuals in fact appear to have ice circulating in their veins and will gladly tell you—if you ask them in so many words—that they have never experienced any emotional distress. They never have any bad days and just don't let stress get to them. So what sort of medication or drug are these folks relying on? The answer is: a large dose of denial.

Of course we all at times have difficult days; in fact these are quite often the norm for the majority of people who seek treatment. But outside my office, I often encounter those macho types who seldom admit willingly to struggling with a challenging situation, feeling, or experience. They tend to cling to the conviction that therapy and medication are only for those weak and misguided souls who are not able to keep their chins up in adversity. When these hard-core Marine types are studied more closely, it turns out that, of course, like you and me, they do in fact have some bad days. But well-designed studies have demonstrated that either they don't view it that way, or else they just don't dwell on these short-term setbacks. Is that a form of Pollyanna optimism, severe denial, or just plain fantasy? I would speculate that this is just another version of the glass-half-full perspective. Those who focus on their successful days and minimize the focus on their problems will at the end of the day experience less stress and a more uplifting mood.

Doctor Pete, I just can't relax!

Many Americans appear to have lost the skill of relaxation. They pay large sums to attend shows, watch sporting events, travel to the Caribbean, etc. While these events may serve as a short-term getaway, the vast majority of their time is spent in a tense and worried mode. Here again, I will let several past patients illustrate this point:

> "Doc, I need you to increase my stimulant. I just can't keep up with the job, the kids, and the housework. Last night at midnight I ran out of gas. You've got to help me out."

> "I have to get out of the hospital today, Doc. If I don't get back to work pronto, my boss will fire me for sure. Then I'll run out of money, and my family will be out on the street." [This, coming from an individual who had attempted to hang himself twenty-four hours before this discussion.]

> "I need a prescription for some Valium. My girlfriend wants me to take her down to Miami Beach. I'm going to have to lie by the pool with her, and you know I'm too hyper to just sit there. Just five or six days would be a big help, Doc."

> "All I want is some kind of medication that will give me a sense of inner peace. What's so difficult about that?"

"I tried to call a few friends after I had that fight with my boyfriend. They didn't pick up, and I just couldn't calm down. I finally decided to take a few pills to try to relax. When that didn't seem to help I took some more. Then I must have gotten kind of confused. After about half an hour I ended up taking the whole bottle. I'm not sure what I was thinking at the time—I just wanted to go to sleep for a while."

Again, most of us know intellectually how to relax, but we seem to have forgotten how to go about it in practice. Or it seems that we have somehow lost the ability to set aside time and energy to do so. We generally view relaxation as a passive behavior, such as watching TV, surfing the Internet, or listening to music. But true relaxation is a fairly consistent response to an actual activity. This tends to differ for any given individual, and it may take some practice, just like any other skill. Of course, Buddhists have a major leg up on the rest of us, with their talents for meditation, as well as their general lack of investment in the material world. For the average Westerner, I often suggest various tools to help in this regard, such as listening to relaxation audiotapes, trying out a few yoga classes, or just setting aside twenty or thirty minutes for basic aerobic activities such as walking.

Perhaps five percent of my patients actually follow through with these suggestions. The vast majority of the other impatient (and unrealistic) souls are convinced that there must be an answer in the convenient form of a tablet or capsule. We will cover this area in more detail in our discussion of the behavioral treatment of mood and anxiety disorders.

Is it just that my situation is depressing, or am I really sick?

This is an area of major difficulty in my field, which has become quite controversial. Many of my patients are quite defensive about their situations. They often present the conviction that anyone in their shoes would share their feelings. Here are some real-life examples, culled from twenty-three years of hard-luck stories:

"If you worked for my boss, you'd be having panic attacks too."

"If my boyfriend would just be faithful to me and stop seeing that other girl, I'd be done with the Zoloft."

"If I just had $10,000, everything would be fine."

"If my son wasn't gay, I wouldn't even be in your office."

"They told me I have a rare condition called scleroderma, which means I'm going to slowly suffocate to death."

"I don't need any more prescriptions, Doc. I just need a new life!"

There are dozens of pressures that could certainly trigger severe anxiety or feelings of loss in just about anyone. As I find myself explaining *ad nauseum*, however, the vast majority of hapless souls with moderate to severe stressors do not end up in my office. Any of the triggers mentioned above, whether vocational, medical, financial, romantic, or familial, is generally not sufficient in and of itself to trigger a full-blown mood disorder. For example, choosing Mussolini as a life partner could raise one's blood pressure to some extent but would not generally lead an Italian woman from the 1940s to develop a severe mood disorder. Even facing the horrors of World War II and the atrocities of the Holocaust did not lead to a consistent depressive reaction on the part of victims, though naturally most survivors of concentration camps emerged with severe post traumatic disorder. Some survivors did, of course ultimately develop severe mood disorders later in life, which would not surprise us, based on the severity of their trauma and the extent of their losses, which often occurred quite early in their fragile lives. But surprisingly, the majority of these victims did not ultimately receive any formal psychiatric treatment and just wanted the freedom to pursue normal lives after their liberation. So, the ones who did develop disorders clearly had a vulnerability that this trauma exposed.

According to the medical model of illness, we postulate that there must be a genetic or biological vulnerability to mood disorders. We are programmed in different ways and thus develop different maladies. When a specific event or trigger exerts enough stress on the individual, this leads to the actual clinical outcome. Thus, some patients under severe stress will tend to develop migraines; others, peptic ulcer disease; and still others, asthma. In my practice, due to the nature of the work that I focus on, I tend to see mood or anxiety disorders. By the same token, most of my colleagues who treat substance abuse disorders find that a spike in the level of stress tends to trigger a relapse or binge. Of course, those with superior coping or stress management skills have a larger margin before their stressors succeed in triggering a clinical disorder.

Why did I get sick (at this time), and what triggered it?

Many patients ask questions about what led them to become depressed or overwhelmed. Some of them present theories that might explain in some reasonably logical fashion how and when their lives changed. However, a large percentage of these unwilling patients are completely at a loss. They might confide in me in the first few visits, "I always thought that I just wasn't the depressed type." Or else, "I'm not the same person I was ten years ago." They are often incredulous that they might be prone to disorders that they might have associated with being "weak," unmotivated, or somehow morally deficient. In many cases they spend much time and energy seeking some sort of elaborate medical evaluation that they think may shed light on their failure to function as expected or that may explain their abrupt sense of panic or hopelessness. My explanation about the complex roots of their specific mood or anxiety disorder in biology, with a specific critical stressors, often meets with blank or disappointed looks.

Why isn't there a test that can tell what's wrong with me?

Many patients are surprised that we currently lack the ability to pinpoint specific imbalances or deficiencies which might lead to their illness.

"What about checking my testosterone? I've heard that having low levels can really affect your mood, plus your energy and motivation."

This very issue, which reflects both patients' and physicians' interest in explaining medical illness in a more precise and biological manner, is currently being debated in the media, due to considerable heated controversy about the new diagnostic manual that was recently released by the American Psychiatric Association. Much of the psychiatric community was hopeful that this highly referenced and authoritative guide to diagnosis and treatment would rely much more heavily than its predecessor on actual objective, scientific data. This might include high-tech radiology procedures, which we refer to as neuroimaging. Or possibly genetic testing, which would ideally shed light on a patient's current disorder, as well as on future vulnerabilities. So the fact that the new manual still relies on a more descriptive, symptom-based approach was viewed as a major disappointment by many of my colleagues, as well as many patients and their families and loved ones.

Why isn't this stuff more scientific? After all, it's 2014!

This debate has primarily targeted the leadership of the association that publishes the manual and that is under scrutiny for each and every change from the prior version. The opposing side has been represented not only by a frustrated public, represented by many advocacy groups, but also by the research branch of the government that focuses on advancing our knowledge of mental health. This entity, the NIMH or National Institute of Mental Health, explicitly challenged the more clinically based writers of the manual to integrate a more research-based nosology, or basis for establishing certain facts and certainties, into their work. The more reasoned view would certainly hope for more progress in developing the tools that help us identify and select treatment for our patients, but it would certainly recognize that the brain is the most complex organ in the world, and this remarkable organ is likely to defy our efforts at understanding for many more centuries. I view this limitation not as a source of frustration but more as a reason for wonder, just as an astronomer marvels at the impossible task of explaining the origin, nature, scale, and boundaries of the universe.

So, when my patient or their well-meaning companions ask these sorts of questions, I am always open to their ideas and concerns. I find it critical to validate their curiosity about the reasons for our limited understanding of the biological basis for psychiatric disorders. As a reasonable alternative, I offer them a widely accepted explanation for what actually triggers an acute episode of illness. This paradigm is founded on what we call the "biopsychosocial model" of psychiatry. Rather than identifying a single cause for a disease, such as streptococcus bacteria which causes strep throat, we have formulated a more integrated and comprehensive understanding of how a disorder evolves. Of course, medical illnesses as well can be viewed in a parallel context, since most of us would agree that simple exposure to a microbe, many of which are already present on our skin, in our gut, or in our throats, is not enough by itself to lead to disease.

Well, you can't pick your genes, can you?

According to this three-part model, which is typically much less complex than that developed by our psychoanalytic predecessors in Vienna, we first identify any biological factors that would predispose a patient to a particular type of disorder. Patients who have relatives with bipolar disorder, addictions, or psychosis are naturally more likely to be afflicted with those—or similar—disorders. We have also learned that there is considerable overlap between the above-mentioned classes of disorders. For example, a man with a history of alcohol dependence might father a daughter who develops intense anxiety instead. Or a woman with a history of bipolar disorder might have a brother with a severe anger problem. Thus the same gene might be expressed differently, depending upon gender or other genetic factors. Additional biological factors could include such direct influences on the brain as excessive thyroid hormone, vitamin deficiency, or, of course, the most common insult to the brain—alcohol or drug intoxication.

I'm really sentimental—I always cry at weddings.

The next trigger we discuss is in the psychological arena, which of course relates to our developmental vulnerabilities. This includes coping skills, defense mechanisms, and the ability to adapt to new challenges. For example, a male with an alcoholic father might have difficulty tolerating any conflict or perceived anger. We all tend to react to various situations in a largely preprogrammed manner, based on our past experiences and interactions. Even though we like to think that we have total control over our actions and responses, the fact is that many—if not most—of our reactions are not consciously mediated. Such minor decisions as which shirt we choose in the morning, all the way up to major decisions such as our choice of a mate, are processed in the unconscious and the areas of the brain that govern irrational behavior. When an event occurs that anyone would view as a setback, the individual's psychological makeup dictates the nature and intensity of the reaction. The patient with poor self-esteem who finds him- or herself abruptly served with divorce papers is likely to respond quite dramatically to this rejection. Another individual who had suffered the loss of his or her mother at an early age would also be expected to have a high risk of a major reaction. This might include such intense feelings as hopelessness, rage, or an overwhelming sadness, perhaps associated with an intense depressive episode. On the other hand, that individual who is more confident and enjoys a range of social support would be expected to experience what we refer to as uncomplicated bereavement. In this case, the rejected spouse would have to work through this loss with a range of feelings but is less likely to develop an incapacitating response.

Those of us who fail to develop trust in others also tend to have a characteristic response to setbacks. A patient who has been neglected or abused by a parent or other important figure will often exhibit a typically magnified response to any real or even perceived rejection. An employee who is downsized is likely to question this decision, and is thus more likely to litigate. A secure individual will be affected by the displacement but will be able to move on more easily, with less likelihood of seeking out a plaintiff attorney or appealing to government agencies.

What about the school of hard knocks?

The last factor that we can outline and understand includes the varied psychosocial pressures that a patient faces. We all deal with a variety of complications, whether we like it or not, though we all have to develop coping skills as we grow up. That being said, most of us would agree that anyone facing financial, vocational, social, or legal setbacks is likely to be stressed and frustrated. The patient with an underlying vulnerability, however, will go on to develop a mood disorder or other psychiatric morbidity.

Biopsychosocial Model

Biological	Psychological	Social
Genetics, medical factors, or exposure to substances	Developmental issues, patterns of reacting or adapting to stress; personality and temperament	Ongoing financial, social, vocational, legal, or other situational pressures vs. supports

Chapter 4

Classifying Psychiatric Disorders

Mood Disorders

Maybe I'm just having a bad day, Doctor Pete.

Many of us wonder whether the increased popularity of psychotherapy and the emergence of such lifestyle drugs as Prozac and Zoloft have led to the overdiagnosis of psychiatric disorders. After all, life is tough, and most of us find that everyday challenges can wear us down. So the bottom line is that we have to be careful in labeling patients with mood disorders. In order to screen for these problems, we have to have an affirmative answer to either (or both) of the following questions:

1. Do I feel distressed or down most of the time?

2. Do I fail to enjoy activities or events in which I would normally find pleasure?

On the other side of the coin, those of us who confidently affirm that they never have a bad day can be clearly proven wrong with a little careful questioning. In this case, in which an individual appears to be in denial about the vagaries of their mood states, the latter question above, related to that person's appreciation or enjoyment of their usual activities, is more relevant.

Why doesn't anyone talk about plain old depression anymore?

This is an interesting topic. For one, many patients with depressed mood see themselves as being potentially bipolar, due to the recent increased focus on this disorder. Most laymen do not realize that patients are usually either at their baseline mood or in a down or depressed mode. They rarely find themselves in a euphoric or revved-up state and thus are classified as having a *unipolar* mood disorder. When I see a patient who tells me that they have periods in which they feel like a million dollars, sometimes that just indicates that they've been suffering for so long that being stable feels quite abnormal to them. It feels really good when you stop hitting your thumb with a hammer. (Don't try this at home.) Plus we can all relate to having a "mood swing" from time to time. Taken to the nth degree, the common household variety mood swing can take on the proportions of full-blown bipolar disorder.

How do I know if I'm bipolar?

As noted above, this has become quite confusing for the layperson over the past several years. Mood disorders include two types—unipolar and bipolar. If you experience only downs and no ups, then you are not bipolar. The confusion did not exist when we used the old-school term for bipolar disorder—"manic depression." Most of us appreciated that our typical outpatient's symptoms of anxiety, frustration, and irritability would not merit a diagnosis of mania. And those of us who periodically spend or drink too much, yell at the wife, or even put a hole in the sheet rock may well be angry and agitated, but, the vast majority of us would not meet the criteria for bipolar unless their irritability lasted for at least seven consecutive days and was associated with other critical symptoms, such as insomnia, anorexia, racing thoughts, etc. However, we all like to explain our impulsive, irrational, or otherwise distasteful behavior in some sort of rational fashion, and this is where the field of psychiatry has often bailed us out—to its discredit. Whenever we find ourselves engaging in self-destructive or impulsive behavior, it can be quite convenient to attribute this to "my ADD" or even bipolar disorder, since there is so much confusion about how to pin down these diagnoses. I hope that the following chart will help establish these disorders more effectively. Keep in mind that a euthymic state is our baseline mood, and that hypomania and dysthymia are less severe forms of mania and depression, respectively. After that, I list the four primary types of mood disorders, from unipolar to bipolar.

	Unipolar	Dysthymia	Bipolar II	Bipolar I	Cyclothymia
Manic				XX	
Hypomanic			XX	XX	XX
Euthymic	XX	XX	XX	XX	XX
Dysthymic	XX	XX	XX	XX	XX
Depressed	XX		XX	XX	

In my line of work, there are many terms for mood disorders, just as Eskimos have many terms for snow. A mild but persistent depressive disorder is called dysthymia. This is a condition that rarely receives medical attention, in which an individual suffers from either a depressed mood or a significant loss of pleasure more than fifty percent of the time. These folks are able to function in most cases. They go to work, raise a family, and take care of their homes, just as the rest of us do, but their quality of life is quite limited much of the time. They tend to feel mildly depressed or sad most of the time. These unfortunate souls often lack pleasure in their usual activities and yet are unable to explain this. They often describe a sense of going through the motions or making plans out of a sense of obligation rather than enjoyment. For the most part, their families and peers would not be able to identify any major concerns, since they can be quite talented at concealing their distress from others. Though they still maintain most of their goals and are able to function at a reasonable level, in the long run their relationships and job prospects become limited. More important, their quality of life is quite compromised, as they might confess to those in their inner circle whom they genuinely trust and rely on.

Another mood disorder could be considered a mild form of bipolar disorder, where people cycle from mild depression to mild manic episodes. This condition is labeled as cyclothymia. These patients are also largely untreated. Compared to dysthymic patients, these more fortunate individuals have the advantage of looking forward to their highs. During hypomanic episodes they can in fact be extremely productive and successful. Some of them opt to forgo treatment when they become aware that they could have both their lows and highs much reduced. Often they come to view a "normal" mood—which we refer to as euthymic—as being subpar, meaning that they tend to perceive any state short of hypomania as being inadequate. They can sometimes make poor decisions when in an elevated mood and can be quite impulsive.

A somewhat more severe form of bipolar disorder, again with less than full-blown manic episodes, is called bipolar type II. This includes both mild to moderate highs, as in cyclothymia, as well as severe lows, which we refer to as major depressive episodes. The highs must last a minimum of seven days, and the lows, at least fourteen days.

I'm thinking faster than I can speak!

Prototypical bipolar disorder, which we term bipolar I in today's nomenclature, includes both full-blown manic and depressive episodes. These patients often times enjoy their highs, which classically include a sense of euphoria and grandiosity. Many of them, however, become irritable and angry when manic, which leads their family, friends, and coworkers either to avoid them or to push them to seek treatment. The difficulty here is that manic patients view themselves as being normal and thus starts to blame everyone around them for the various complications that result from their impulsive and irrational behavior. If they drive thirty miles per hour over the speed limit and rear-end another vehicle, this is undoubtedly because the other driver jammed on his brakes. If patients engage in extramarital affairs, this is in fact payback because their spouses must have had several affairs in the past year. These conclusions are not based on reality, but on patients' own brand of logic. In general such patients are quite skilled at justifying their behavior by making use of a form of twisted thinking. If the manic patient errs in investing a large sum of money in an investment that ultimately fails, leading to a monumental loss, they may explain that the CEO of the company was somehow being paid off by the mafia to drive the business into the ground. If he decides to leave his family, cash in his 401K, and fly out to Vegas for the weekend, that is because he has figured out how to count cards, even with four decks in play on the blackjack table.

A large percentage of these patients do in fact become psychotic, which might take the form of a paranoid delusion—e.g., that they are being cheated on. Others might start to experience hallucinations, though often they are unlikely to disclose these symptoms since they recognize the odd nature of these events. In my experience the psychotic material is an extension of the unconscious feelings that they cannot tolerate.

For example, one female patient I treated presented with the delusion that her husband was Charles Manson, which led to her decision to flee from the home. During treatment this belief resolved, to the extent that she dutifully decided to return to her marriage. She described her husband as more principled and spiritual than she was and criticized herself as having erred by not following his every wish over the past two years of their short relationship. During her two-week stay in the hospital, we were able to observe several formal and informal sessions in which the couple interacted. To our surprise, it was quite clear that he treated her in a controlling, condescending, and demeaning fashion. She was discharged and returned to their apartment, even though the treatment team found him in fact quite unworthy of her. We were thus pleased to learn that just two weeks after her release from the hospital she had summarily packed his bags and asked him to leave the apartment. She had become uncomfortable with the conflictual state of finding herself angry and confused about the relationship that she had somehow chosen for herself. Once this conflict became less intense, she was able to view her husband not as an evil murderer, but instead simply as an unpleasant and mean-spirited individual who had no legitimate business being her husband. If we had confronted this delusion early in treatment, the patient would have protested vociferously and perhaps even have started to view us, her treating doctors, as part of some vast conspiracy designed to force her to return to her intolerable marriage. So we have to recognize that the presenting delusion always has some basis in reality, meaning that every psychotic symptom has a rationale.

I'm the only one who's on the ball!

While most depressed patients will tell you that they feel sad or lack enjoyment in most of their usual activities, manic patients will tell you that they are doing well, thank you very much. Even though they might have just told their boss to sit on a brass tack or asked their neighbor's spouse to elope with them to the South Pacific, they view themselves as 100 percent focused and reasonable. If you take the time to listen to their often convoluted and scattered explanations, such patients can justify any and all sorts of outrageous and even dangerous decisions.

This is to say that they lack insight into their illness and for this reason fail to see themselves as ill. Most bipolar patients are either compelled to seek treatment on an involuntary basis, or they decide to cooperate during a depressive episode when they are clearly suffering and can accept input from psychiatric clinicians.

Manic mind, manic body

The other important point is that these disorders are also medically based, meaning that the patient has many physiological symptoms in addition to psychological ones. The vast majority of patients invariably have difficulty with many physiological functions, such as sleep, appetite, libido, concentration, energy, etc. When their mood starts to cycle into a manic or depressive episode, many of them have dramatic and measurable changes in their blood pressure, serum glucose, basal metabolism, or other significant functions. When these physical symptoms coexist with the negative thoughts and poor self-esteem described above, this indicates a clinical mood disorder.

When you hear hoof beats, don't think "zebras."

Even though many patients are concerned that they may be misdiagnosed, one good tactic is to play the odds. Unipolar depression is much more common than the bipolar form, though when we are treating a younger person, the latter disorder needs to be considered. In older patients, especially with triggers such as bereavement, chronic medical illness, isolation, etc., unipolar depression is much more prevalent. If a high school student is failing his classes but tends to fall asleep in school because he goes to sleep at two o'clock in the morning, I would say that he has a basic sleep-deprivation issue, rather than attention deficit disorder.

What about if my teenage son just doesn't seem motivated? Is he depressed?

This is truly the $64,000 question, which is usually posed by the frustrated parent, spouse, sibling, or child of the unmotivated individual. If only there were a medication to get us moving, to push us to take out the garbage, do our dreaded paperwork, weed the garden, start that diet that we've been pondering for decades, and take on all those other tasks, the pharmaceutical industry would be in clover. This is probably the second most common issue that is raised in my office, behind only the issue of dealing with stress or anxiety (see below). Many folks are able to spend time with friends, engage in various recreational activities, eat with gusto, sleep like a baby, and generally pass their time in relative comfort. They have one failing, however: they don't do any actual work. This might be sustainable for the Prince of Wales, but even he has to have some kind of mission to keep the queen and the press from complaining about his lack of nobility.

Those of us who are not followed by paparazzi and photographed for *People* magazine, however, tend to follow a basic principle: we do what we have to do. If someone tells me that they have been paying their son's rent, car lease, credit card bills, etc. I would not be surprised if that prodigal son failed to report for duty every morning. As a corollary, an associated principle is that many of us will do whatever we can get away with. Accordingly, if the above-mentioned son is able to extract funds from his father and evade any gainful employment, then why should we expect him to pound the pavement and apply for low-paying, unglamorous positions?

Common Anxiety Disorders

Anxiety disorders are also to a large extent misunderstood. Most commonly we see patients who are constantly tense and worried. This affects them both emotionally and physically, just as mood disorders do. They notice tight muscles, increased sweating, tension headaches, stomach upset, insomnia, anorexia, you name it. This ultimately leads to a state of withdrawal, since the afflicted individual tends to respond by attempting to "chill out"—i.e., lying on the sofa, flipping on the TV, pouring a drink, etc. This pattern unfortunately tends to backfire, leading to more worrying and physical tension. Chronic tension actually wears down your energy reserves.

How could you relax when the universe is expanding?

We refer to this syndrome as generalized anxiety disorder, which is measurably more common in the present than 50 years ago. This sense of tension and unease affects a patient most of the time and leads to consistent physical complaints.

Generalized anxiety represents a significant disorder that merits detection and treatment. While in general no one ends up in the emergency room due to this demoralizing condition, primary care physicians spend much of their day dealing with the myriad concerns and issues that these frustrated and challenging patients present. Due to the variety of seemingly unconnected issues, the doctor's quest to link all the symptoms in a coherent fashion to one specific disorder is generally fruitless. The eventual outcome is that the patient ends up with assorted—often ineffective—recommendations and therapies. Once the clinician realizes that the presenting symptoms are all stress-related, the diagnosis becomes more visible.

But the doctor says it's all in your head!

The concern with this approach is that we might start to view legitimate disorders as "psychosomatic," meaning that we write off the patient's complaints as triggered by stress. For this reason I would caution clinicians who attribute their anxious patient's symptoms to psychiatric conditions to remember that patients with anxiety and related conditions can also develop medical problems. It would be foolish to determine that a disorder is psychologically based prior to taking a medical history and doing an examination.

What if the sky really is falling down?

Panic attacks are more insidious. They occur only occasionally, last for fairly short periods of time, but, like earthquakes, leave an indelible memory. They can last from minutes to hours but feel like an eternity. The sensation is of intense fear, along with arousal—pounding heart, sweaty palms, quavering voice, shortness of breath, butterflies in the stomach, dizziness, and fear of fainting. To sum it up, envision the most terrified feeling that you've ever experienced in your life, and imagine feeling that way several times per day or week. Welcome to the world of panic disorder.

Patients often live in constant fear of sustaining another attack, which they fear might occur in the car and cause them to lose control and drive into a tree. (This doesn't actually occur, in case you were wondering.) Or perhaps an attack will happen at work, during an important meeting, from which the patient will abruptly feel compelled to exit. Other patients suspect that they might faint in the middle of a date or job interview. Still others become dizzy, generally due to hyperventilating, and are convinced that they will pass out and fall down. These events tend to evoke a sense of impending doom, in addition to uncomfortable physical experiences that might replicate an asthmatic or cardiac event. "I just couldn't breathe." "I felt like my heart was going a mile a minute." "I thought it was the big one." Many of these patients are initially evaluated in the emergency room and undergo considerable testing, since they fear dying during an episode. Even though most of them are quite young, they are convinced that there must be a medical explanation for their misery. When the well-intentioned emergency room physician informs the patient that he or she is medically stable with no clear-cut disorders, the physician's remarks often trigger frustration rather than relief.

> "Doc, you don't understand! I could feel my heart skipping beats. I could have dropped dead!"

> "I suddenly felt all hot and cold. I think it had something to do with my new birth control pill."

"I had nothing to be worried about. I was just watching a ball game and then all of a sudden I couldn't even breathe. I think it was some kind of asthma attack."

"That emergency room doctor spent maybe ten minutes with me. He must have missed something. I'm going to see a specialist."

Many individuals will insist on more testing, second opinions, and even medications that they might not truly benefit from. Based on the severity of their symptoms, they are unable to accept that they have no specific medical diagnosis. For this reason it is critical that primary care and emergency room staff become familiar with this disorder in order to minimize unnecessary testing and clarify the patient's concerns as fully and effectively as possible.

This disorder, known as panic disorder, can often lead to increasing efforts to avoid any potential setting that might either trigger a panic attack or that might be difficult to escape from in the event of a perceived emergency. These patients are thus at high risk of developing the extremely treatment-resistant syndrome known as agoraphobia. They may start to limit their range of activities to the point that they might decide to remain at home, which becomes a comfort zone. I once treated a patient who had been missing for twenty years and who in fact was thought to have died. In reality he stayed in his home and had no contact with any neighbors, friends, or extended relatives for over two decades. Talk about a Rip Van Winkle experience!

Step on the crack, break your mother's back!

Other anxiety disorders are commonly discussed but less commonly seen in practice. Those of us who speak of coworkers with OCD are generally referring to a personality style that evokes Felix Unger of *The Odd Couple*. This includes a tendency to dwell excessively on trivial details and many other perfectionist traits that ultimately interfere with one's ability to function in the real world. The actual disorder that we speak of in a clinical setting is the syndrome that includes intrusive thoughts or obsessions, along with compulsive behaviors driven by fear. This encompasses behaviors such as checking, cleaning, washing, counting, etc. The disorder that many commonly refer to as OCD is actually correctly classified as obsessive compulsive personality disorder. This would be properly viewed as a longstanding adaptation, which tends to be a lifelong condition, rather than an acute disorder. This adaptation would be welcomed in a cardiac surgeon, accountant, or financial planner—at least in their professional capacity. At home the surgeon's families and friends would clearly be alienated if he or she spent hours carving a steak in the middle of a dinner party. The accountant's family would be aggravated if he or she demanded every receipt from the supermarket in order to balance the checkbooks.

Shell shock, survivor's syndrome, soldier's heart, and most recently ...

Posttraumatic disorders are widely discussed but are in fact not common, except in veterans, refugees, and victims of violent crime. This disorder, which falls on the spectrum of anxiety disorders, entails several manifestations of severe anxiety, including hypervigilance, nightmares, flashbacks, and severe reactions to triggers that bring up memories of the traumatic event. These disorders also can be viewed as a form of OCD in that the patient experiences intrusive, distressing thoughts and images that are chronic and often difficult to treat.

Psychotic Disorders

This group is in fact quite limited and less common, though of course the impact of psychosis—essentially, losing touch with reality—can be quite devastating. This includes schizophrenia, which has several subtypes; a variation in which there is a marked mood component, as well as psychotic features, called schizoaffective disorder; and brief reactive psychosis. With psychosis, we generally expect to see longstanding, pervasive, and progressive social and vocational difficulties, along with characteristic behavioral changes. Fortunately these patients tend to respond quite well, given appropriate treatment, support, and resources. The fact that many of them experience dramatic symptoms such as voices, bizarre delusions, paranoid thinking, etc. is generally less important in the long run than the more disabling functional deficits. These deficits, which tend to precede the onset of psychotic behavior, and respond much less consistently to treatment, include lack of motivation, difficulty focusing, social isolation, and apathy. Many severely ill patients are able to function successfully in the workplace in spite of their delusions, as long as they are motivated to overcome—or can simply learn to tolerate—these symptoms. The more chronically disabled patients are those who deny any voices or paranoia but have a so-called "negative syndrome" in which they fail to maintain any goals and essentially withdraw from the world. Even though only one percent of the population is afflicted with schizophrenia, the financial, emotional, vocational, and societal impact of this condition is enormous. Most of the progress I have witnessed over the past twenty-three years in my profession has mainly consisted of improved and earlier detection, more effective but still quite limited medication interventions, and increased acceptance and understanding of how this illness affects so many unfortunate individuals.

Where did all these homeless people come from? Why are the jails so overcrowded?

On the negative side, I have also witnessed the repercussions of our efforts to move toward an outpatient model of treatment, which can be quite fragmented and frustrating in its actual execution. The promise of comprehensive treatment for what we refer to as chronic and persistent mental illness has never been fulfilled. This approach would have included intensive case management, family therapy, outreach services, and aggressive social and vocational rehabilitation, all of which would supplement progress in the understanding and psychiatric care of these disorders, which include schizophrenia, resistant depressive and bipolar disorders, developmental disorders such as autism, and severe impulse control disorders. The grand plans outlined by John F. Kennedy in the '60s have largely been dismantled over the past fifty years. The results? A substantial minority of prison inmates with mental illness, with only modest access to treatment, at best. A growing number of homeless people, also untreated. A broken trail of patients who drift from one short period of stabilization to another, with no true continuity of care. Thousands of families who are witnessing their loved ones deteriorate and fall through the cracks, with no true recourse other than the courts.

The reason for these failings? This topic could certainly occupy the rest of this guide, but I will keep it brief:

1) Harsh economic measures, such as closing down countless outpatient and inpatient programs, which save in the short term but ultimately cost us much more.

2) A focus on patients' rights that prevents us from treating patients who are unwilling to accept their illness. As with mania, the lack of insight into one's illness is a cardinal feature of schizophrenia. This results in a situation in which we are able to treat patients only when they become dangerous to themselves or others, or are blatantly incapable of caring for themselves.

3) Society's discomfort with these confusing and intimidating disorders, along with the stigma and fear that arises when the occasional violent crime or mass murder is committed by an individual who has undergone some form of psychiatric care.

The reality is that the vast majority of patients are destined to be victims of crimes, rather than perpetrators. Since society fails to take them seriously, they are usually either unwilling or unable to exact justice in a court of law when they are wronged.

What about the Woodstock generation?

Of course, as noted in the initial process of diagnosing these disorders, many family members wonder if their loved one, who is often college age and thus potentially exposed to many mind-altering substances, may have what we refer to as a "drug-induced" psychosis. This condition is triggered by substantial and chronic use of a stimulant, though hallucinogens are also implicated in many cases. Some of the most agitated and paranoid individuals that I have treated were long-time abusers of crack cocaine, PCP, or amphetamines. Of course, these disorders tend to subside with time as long as the patient abstains from further use. It also is important to note that only a small percentage of individuals who use marijuana, cocaine, LSD, or painkillers develop an acute psychiatric disorder. Many families cling to the idea that their son or daughter's inappropriate behavior was triggered by an episode of substance abuse. In this case, naturally, they would be relieved of the fear that their child might suffer from a severe and persistent psychiatric condition. While I do not rush to disabuse them of this conviction, I also tend to encourage them to focus on both a plan to work toward substance-free living in addition to ongoing treatment for their psychiatric disorder. Should the disorder resolve with time and sobriety, then of course the patient is free to forgo ongoing treatment, provided that they refrain from using any alcohol or drugs.

But my son is only sick because he had a really high fever when he was three!

The second common concern that patients present to my office is that they might have an underlying medical disorder that has led to a change in their mood or functional status. Medical conditions that trigger psychosis have certainly been documented, especially in the days of untreated syphilis, but they are quite uncommon in this era of modern medicine. Of course severe neurological injuries are associated with clear-cut changes in behavior, some of which can at times masquerade as a mood or other purely psychiatric disorder. For example, I once was called to evaluate a young man for a depressive disorder. He had sustained leaking of an artery in the brain, known as a cerebral aneurysm. Once the defective vessel was successfully clipped off by a neurosurgeon, the staff and family noticed a dramatic change in this unfortunate patient's demeanor. A formerly animated and gregarious individual, he was withdrawn and laconic, with monosyllabic responses to questions. He lacked interest in visiting with friends, failed to shave or take care of his personal appearance, and generally appeared detached. He denied any depressed feelings, however, and simply found that the world was moving too fast for him. He thus had a different experience based on the injuries that he sustained from his intracranial bleeding, as well as the damage to the parts of the brain that lost blood flow once the offending artery was no longer providing circulation.

Impulse Control Disorders

This group includes those sins of commission that we read about in the daily papers or see on the six o'clock news. Many individuals appear stable from a psychiatric perspective and do not voice any complaints, but nonetheless have difficulty regulating their impulses. When placed in a specific situation, they lack the ability to manage their behavior in a rational or measured manner. Of course we all suffer from this type of disorder at various points in our lives. We might spend too much at the outlet stores. Or we might take the bait and engage in a verbal altercation at the Thanksgiving table, even though our children are present. Or a promising young congressman might succumb to the impulse to send compromising photos to a young admirer, even though he knows full well that this could easily derail his entire career, his marriage, and his family life. As human beings we are plagued with a series of wishes and urges, which Freud described as being driven by the pleasure center of the brain—the id. Some of us are more successful in slowing down and nipping these urges in the bud, based on either:

- The ability to delay gratification, or

- The understanding that a short-term pleasurable experience could lead to a longer-term form of discomfort, including shame, guilt, or unpleasant consequences that we are not willing to endure.

In the case of either impulse control disorders, addictions, or other compulsive behaviors, the ability to process or fully think through and intercept an urge to perform unwanted or inappropriate actions is somehow impaired. Either the impulse is just too intense, or the part of the brain that maps out decisions and their possible repercussions is not as highly developed or active as in those fortunate folks who act in a more measured and rational fashion. The patient I describe next demonstrates what we refer to as intermittent explosive disorder.

A thirty-five-year-old white male was admitted to the inpatient psychiatric unit. He had been selling cars and was convinced that his manager had shorted him six thousand dollars. After a brief and intense argument, he started his car and drove in the direction of the dealership floor. As the other salesmen took cover, he drove the car through the glass entrance doors into the showroom. As the glass shattered all around him, he yelled at his manager, "Are you going to pay up now?"

Needless to say, this stunt either tends to land you in jail or in an emergency room, which he opted for. The diagnosis was tentatively bipolar disorder, though he appeared quite calm and presentable when I saw him the following day. He was somewhat embarrassed about his loss of control but not overly remorseful. For a moment I thought he would fit in better in the local jail. He didn't seem especially impulsive or unstable. When one of our nurses explained the smoking policy (no on-unit smoking; forty-eight hours until he might receive a pass to leave the unit for short smoke breaks with a group), however, he again started to become agitated. He demanded to leave and began to pound the entrance door with his fists. We started to prepare for a team effort to persuade him to take a sedative, and called security in the event that he became assaultive. Fortunately, at that point his mother appeared for visiting hours. Within thirty seconds he was transformed from Mr. Hyde into Dr. Jekyll, with a sheepish apology to the staff, prompted by his mother. (As a side note, he did ultimately receive his full commission of roughly $6,000. Unfortunately for him, the cost of repairing the front of the dealership was $8,000, so his anger and impulsive behavior ended up costing him $2,000 of his hard-earned money.)

So how does an addiction really differ from any other impulse control disorder?

This is a good question. In my view, an addiction is really just an example of an impulse control disorder. It just so happens that the action in this case pertains to the use of alcohol or drugs. On the other hand, many of the effects of addiction result from direct exposure of the brain to the substance in question. The alcoholic who has already had one drink is quite different from the one who is just thinking about that drink. Should that individual successfully avoid people, places, and things associated with alcohol, as well as that substance itself, they are much more likely to remain sober. In the same vein, a gambler who avoids any context with casinos, racetracks, poker parties, etc. is also more likely to avoid setbacks in his or her ability to refrain from gambling.

What about bad habits, like biting my nails? Is that am impulse control disorder?

Many of us are guilty of picking up various "bad habits," which we engage in, in spite of the negative impact they have on us or on others around us. These are activities that are not rewarding in and of themselves but that are difficult to refrain from because they have present for extended periods of time in which these behaviors become difficult to dislodge. Many of them are exacerbated by stress but often exist even during times of calm. Though many of these activities bring on embarrassment and social scorn, they can be quite persistent and difficult to treat. One example is a mouthful—trichotillomania. This involves the compulsive pulling of one's hair. Many patients afflicted with this disorder end up quite mortified, with bald spots on their head or missing eyebrows. Other more common behaviors include picking at or biting one's nails, repetitive blinking, checking one's cell phone, etc. There are many successful behavioral treatments for these conditions, but the patient has to commit to making a change in his or her behavior, in addition to working on stress management techniques, in order to have a successful outcome.

So what's wrong with overdoing it once in a while?

Naturally there is no harm in having an occasional urge to argue with the boss, or to lock one's teenager in the library when they bring home a poor report card. It is only when one fails to resist an unhealthy impulse that the disorder emerges. Every day every one of us has impulses of all varieties—to buy a new car, to change careers, to tell our boss to jump in a lake, to spank our teenager for failing to take out the garbage, and so on. But as I point out to many of my patients, having an impulse does not force us to act on it. This ability to control our impulses is lacking in patients who fall into this category. This includes a variety of troublesome behaviors, such as gambling, shoplifting, pulling out one's hair, and the more intimidating diagnosis of "intermittent explosive disorder." One theory behind these disorders explains that the command center of the rain, which is located in the prefrontal cortex behind the forehead, might be underactive in certain control centers. These areas serve a veto or inhibitory role in the brain. When they fail to light up in a situation when an individual is tempted to make a sudden and poorly thought out decision, the diagnosis of an impulse control disorder may come into play. Unfortunately these disorders can be quite resistant to treatment and thus are often addressed under the auspices of our legal or penal system.

The impulse control disorders do not include deviant sexual behavior, which has its own place in our nomenclature and is beyond the scope of this discussion. Nor does it include addictive behavior, though of course one could easily view this as a variant form of impulsive behavior.

Addiction Disorders

We have dealt with these disorders for thousands of years, ever since the discovery of fermentation, tobacco, opium, and coca leaves. Most of us are able to regulate our use of these agents fairly easily, despite the rewarding nature of these substances. But unfortunately about 15 percent of us develop an intense preoccupation with them, which has negative consequences. Rather than the old-school view of addiction, which viewed it as a weakness or character flaw, we now view this behavior as medically based with a major genetic component. Since we cannot choose or modify our genes (as of yet, in any case), it behooves us to be vigilant about our Achilles heel or areas of vulnerability. Many patients become hooked on their drug of choice after only one use. And we all know smokers who are bright, educated, and responsible individuals. So these disorders are not afflictions of the weak or immoral, but instead a hardwired response to extremely compelling chemical interactions in the brain.

I'd rather fight than switch!

You might have heard of the experiments in which rats or monkeys starve to death in the throes of cocaine intoxication. The substance becomes more appealing or compelling than food, or even life itself. For those of us who are fortunate enough to lack this vulnerability or never to have been exposed to potential hazards, this may appear to be a willful, conscious decision on the part of the addict. But just as I tend to obsess about food if I haven't had a lunch break by two or three o'clock, addicts spend their day dwelling on their craving for their particular substance.

Following is one patient's account of her experience with alcohol addiction:

> "In my mind, just a little drink will help me cope with my life. I was driving home, and my disease spoke to me. I heard, 'You can go get a bottle—it will take the stress away.' Five miles from my house I was finally determined to buy the bottle. I knew it was wrong, but I didn't care. I drank for about two months, and I became more depressed. Finally I decided to get help and I found a doctor I could share my pain with."

While at least at the onset, the odds of successfully treating an addict are quite daunting, we are fortunate to have a reasonable variety of medical tools to help these folks in their quest for sobriety. The discussion about these agents will follow in the section on treatments. Clearly, education is a critical piece of the puzzle as well. If a patient is not aware that the average ex-smoker will require seven or eight discrete attempts prior to quitting for good, he or she will tend to become frustrated and give up after one or two efforts. If the patient is not aware of the availability of several tools to facilitate this process, both medication-based and alternative, they may face an uphill battle. So, in this case, a little bit of knowledge can go a long way.

I would also suspect that in the next few decades we will learn much more about the biological underpinnings of addiction, since the way we respond to various agents varies so broadly between individuals. The precise substance that makes one of us euphoric might trigger sadness or paranoia in another. Patients with attention deficit disorder tend to feel calmer with stimulants like amphetamines, while most of us would become more energized and even agitated.

Personality Disorders, or, "You should really be seeing my wife, Doctor Pete. She's the crazy one."

This is an area in which there is much interest and casual labeling, but also much confusion. As noted above, we tend to adapt to the world in many different ways in a manner that works for us. Those of us who feel neglected or not cared for tend to focus on meeting our own needs, to the exclusion of others', and we refer to this condition as a narcissistic disorder. Those of us who tend to have very intense feelings, unstable relationships, and a constant state of turmoil often emerge with a borderline personality disorder. Those who are chronically fearful of being judged or rejected by their peers develop avoidant personality disorders. Individuals who are unable to function independently or make decisions without relying excessively on others are classified as having a dependent personality disorder.

Features of Personality Disorders

1) The patient sees his or her dysfunctional behavior as normal.

2) The patient's pattern of behavior represents a longstanding adaptation that allows the individual to minimize his or her exposure to conflicts.

3) When others become critical of the patient's maladaptive behavior, he or she finds fault with them, rather than accepting their point of view.

4) Only when the patient's adaptation fails, leading to a severe crisis, does the patient consider seeking professional help.

5) Because these disorders are quite entrenched, their treatment usually takes one of two forms. Either it is extremely short-term and focused, which requires working through a crisis and allowing the patient to resume his or her usual behavior, meaning that the therapist reinforces the patient's usual coping skills, or the therapist must devote considerable time and effort to helping the patient modify and restructure his or her maladaptive behavior.

Based on the first criterion outlined above, in most cases these patients are generally not interested in psychiatric treatment. This results from the fact that they are not usually in distress and can often function quite well, to a point. Thus there is no basis for identifying them as mentally ill. They have characteristic patterns in their interactions with other people and see the world through their own lens. For the most part, their coping skills allow them to succeed in their own fashion, to a certain extent. It is only when their usual adaptation fails them, or when the outside world gives them harsh and negative feedback, that they become frustrated and overwhelmed. When they show up in my office, often under duress, they present a series of setbacks or repetitive negative outcomes in their work or interpersonal lives. One patient stated:

> "I didn't want any treatment until my life became unmanageable. My stress level was over the edge, and I saw no way out."

It's not me, it's you!

For people with personality disorders, a major problem in their interactions either at home or at work can trigger severe anxiety. These patients usually still view their own behavior as appropriate and thus often rationalize their setbacks. Instead of accepting responsibility for an interpersonal conflict, they generally blame others. So rather than rationalizing, the terms "blaming" or "displacing" might prove more accurate. Typically, these aggrieved folks will inform me that "my wife is the one who should be in your office, since she's the problem." Or else, "I'd be doing fine at work if my boss wasn't such an incompetent nincompoop." In general they view the world with a highly critical eye, since most of us do not conform to their model of how things should work. Their preferred role is Monday morning quarterback or frustrated executive. Due to their tendency to blame others for throwing a wrench into the works, rather than being accountable themselves, they tend to seek treatment only under duress. Once in my office, they generally present a litany of complaints about various people and events that have conspired to limit their success in various nefarious ways.

Since these personality styles are chronic and serve a purpose for the individual, people with personality disorders usually put up a great deal of resistance to any attempt to modify these adaptations. In addition, these patients tend to excel at placing blame on others, and take responsibility for conflicts or problems only reluctantly if at all. Another obstacle arises when we attempt to take away someone's customary coping tools. Most often they will naturally protest and fail to cooperate, with a focus on making other people change, rather than themselves. They also share a tendency to bolt from treatment once the crisis situation is averted. To complicate matters, we have very few tried and true treatments for these longstanding disorders that would help in a short-term time frame compatible with today's health care models and economics. These disorders can therefore be difficult to address. The most logical course of action is often to reinforce the patient's usual coping strategies and work toward a compromise with the offended person. In fact, most successful outcomes involve educating and supporting the individuals who are affected by the identified patient, who usually has limited or no interest in treatment or change. Modifying one's adaptation to the world is a Herculean task that would take extensive work on the part of the patient, as well as intensive resources on the part of our healthcare system.

Chapter 5

The Medical Basis
for Psychiatric Treatment

How do all these problems respond to medication?

This is certainly a valid question. If the workings of the brain are so complex, and our treatment options so limited, how could we expect to make a dent in major psychological disorders with medication? At present our understanding of the chemical and electrical activity of the brain is so rudimentary that it turns out that many of our current treatments were discovered serendipitously. In other words, scientists were using medication for entirely different purposes but then found that many agents had a significant impact on behavior. For example, Thorazine, an antipsychotic, was initially studied as an antihistamine. Depakote, a mood stabilizer, was used as a solvent for other medications when it was found to have a positive impact on its own. Newer agents are usually identified in a somewhat more sophisticated manner— by seeking out compounds that have a similar side-effect profile. Unfortunately this limits us to a large extent to imposing the same adverse effects in order to reap the same rewards. Another study utilizes an animal model, which relies on helping the study animals tolerate various forms of stress. In reducing the subject's reactions to various negative stimuli, this approach risks reducing the individual's reactions to and appreciation of a positive or rewarding event.

So this approach is clearly a double-edged sword. Many patients do in fact relate that their lows are not as low a few weeks after starting on medication. They often, however, find themselves in a state of relative apathy that potentially robs them of much of the joy they might experience in the course of their day. This outcome actually evokes the historical underside of my field—the past reliance on sedation, chemical strait jackets, and even surgical lobotomies to manage behavioral disorders, most of whose victims were not ostensibly aggressive and did not require such heavy-handed interventions.

Many patients come in with the expectation that I will have access to a high-tech blood test or imaging study, such as an MRI of the brain, which will shed light on their diagnosis and treatment. This is where the crystal ball comes in. While most of us would accept that the brain is quite a complex organ, some frustrated individuals appear to be convinced that modern science has it all figured out. We toss around theories about serotonin, dopamine, etc., which help us feel more confident in our work. Ultimately, however, we have to acknowledge that most of our knowledge is merely empirical, meaning that, while we have effective treatments, we have very little understanding of how these disorders emerge and how our treatments work. The important point is that treatment does work.

Why can't he just do a blood test to see if I need more dopamine or perhaps some more turkey in my diet?

"But what is this stuff doing to my brain?"

"What is the mechanism of action for treating a depressive disorder?"

We have several approaches for understanding mood and anxiety disorders. Initially we were fixated on norepinephrine, which serves a fight-or-flight response. This chemical serves to activate the alarm center in the brain, which tracks and responds to the level of pressures one is facing. Treatments which appeared to reduce to impact of this process were also successful in addressing many mood disorders. These medications included the oldest type of mood elevating medications,

MAO inhibitors, as well as the second generation of medications, tricyclic antidepressants. We found that these medications were helpful with mood, but were difficult to employ on a frequent basis. The former group, MAO inhibitors, pose a significant danger if combined with certain foods or medications and thus have been eschewed by many of my colleagues in spite of their effectiveness. The second group, tricyclic antidepressants, can affect a patient's blood pressure or cardiac conduction. In addition, many patients disliked the significant side effects which occur especially at higher doses.

Proposed Mechanism of Antidepressants

Many well-educated individuals have the misconception that we actually have a crystal-clear and comprehensive understanding of how the brain works. They are convinced that we have mapped out the billions of neurons in the brain and their operations. This involves billions of electrical impulses, as well as thousands of chemicals, of which we currently understand only a smattering. Often they wonder whether there is some dietary issue or just some simple vitamin deficiency. They appear crestfallen when I try to explain that modern science is just not up to the Star Trek level at present. Even in the medical or surgical worlds, many disorders are poorly understood and are treated with only partially effective or controversial methods. In fact, as many as half of patients with imposing symptoms such as chest pain, headaches, dizziness, vertigo etc. are never formally diagnosed. That is to say that, in spite of extensive testing and examination over a period of time, the medical team is unable to pin down the specific condition responsible for the presenting complaints. The good news is that modern medicine is quite good at ruling out serious and life-threatening conditions and that most of the unexplained conditions resolve with time and 'supportive interventions (meaning a couple of Tylenols and a good night's rest).

A Revolutionary Treatment in Search of a Disease

The nervous system is so complex and interconnected that any mood-altering chemical tends to affect many different areas in the brain. We generally find that a medication that helps boost your mood generally reduces your level of anxiety as well. And of course once the pharmaceutical executives realized that, their marketing teams went into overdrive. Suddenly there were many new reasons to prescribe these medications. First they decided to study Prozac for panic attacks. Then for OCD. Next for premenstrual dysphoric disorder. (That included repackaging the old Prozac capsule in a pretty pink and lavender shell, to be more appealing to the fair sex.) Then the business model argued for an extremely broad market—they decided to target milder forms of depression, such as dysthymia. Traditionally these low-grade disorders were treated by therapists or perhaps even by the individual's usual support system. Some experts would even advise a wait-and-see approach, since mood can improve with time and support in many cases. This pattern where the problem resolves without any formal intervention would be akin to the use of an antibiotic for a nasty head cold—by the time the patient starts on the medication, he or she is already on the mend anyway. But the pharmaceutical industry would not want us to take any chances, based on the possibility that the mild disorder could progress into a severe episode. And this was just the beginning … what about the life-style indications? When this blockbuster was launched, many hoped that these medications would help solve the longstanding quagmire of compulsive eating. So of course Eli Lilly embarked on weight-loss trials, with modest success but nothing definitive. In spite of some promising data, it turned out that, of the multitude of factors that might lead to overeating, only a limited number respond to treatment with serotonin-based agents. Then many clinicians hoped for a safe and nonaddictive approach to boosting one's motivation and allaying one's inhibitions. This also appeared successful for a period of time, but any benefit generally fizzled out in a matter of weeks. So we had some disappointments over the years, though in my opinion the major impact of Prozac has yet to be understood.

It seems that the chemical in question, serotonin, helps to regulate the primitive parts of the brain that govern fear and the so-called "fight-or-flight" response. Those of us who develop anxiety disorders appear to have overly active serotonin transmission, leading to a state of almost constant vigilance. The serotonin-based anxiety medications help to reduce the level of sensitivity to this transmitter. So via this mechanism, we find that Prozac and other similar medications help modulate or tone down our response to perceived dangers or threats.

Those of us who are tempted to get up from our chairs and head for the hills when our bosses make a disparaging comment are more likely to stick it out. Those of us who are tempted to argue with our teenagers when they criticize our taste in neckties or sports cars have more success keeping it zipped.

How do I fix my chemical imbalance?

Many scientists have postulated that those with mood or anxiety disorders have an underlying imbalance of various chemicals in the brain, just as patients with diabetes have difficulty adjusting their level of insulin and other critical hormones. Using this line of reasoning, many patients believe there must be some sort of supplement or dietary change that would correct this imbalance so that formal treatment would be unnecessary. Many patients have in fact sought out this solution, with the presumption that we have a full understanding of the brain's chemical and electrical activity. Unfortunately, this conviction is quite far from the reality of neural science. Most honest researchers will confess that, while we have made considerable progress, we understand only roughly 20 per cent of what actually transpires either to maintain a healthy mood or, alternatively, to trigger a mood or anxiety disorder. In my view we could conceive of a mood disorder in which important regions in the brain are less active than usual, leading to a depressed state. The converse hypothesis proposes that, in a cycling or manic disorder, areas of the brain are overly active, leading to mood swings. These theories have in fact been substantiated by what we call functional imaging studies, which measure the extent of metabolism of glucose in various parts of the brain.

Further evidence of this model follows from our experience with medications. Depressive disorders respond to activating agents, which increase the level of certain critical chemicals, which we call neurotransmitters. Cycling disorders respond to agents—generally from the class of anti-seizure medications—that instead slow down electrical transmissions in the brain.

Another, less developed, model that is helpful in understanding the chemistry of mood disorder revolves around excitatory and inhibitory chemicals. The use of the former class is less established, even in depressive disorders, since excessive excitatory input tends to increase one's level of anxiety or agitation. The latter class is widely preferred, which goes back to our discussion about sedatives. The primary chemical that helps calm brain activity, GABA, for short, is the basis for all of our sedatives, including alcohol, and many antiseizure agents used for bipolar or impulse control disorders. All these medications have an impact on the GABA receptors in the brain, which turns down the amplitude of activity in many important areas in the brain. The downside of this effect is that, though we feel calmer and more "together," we are operating on less than full capacity. Increasing levels of GABA can make us sleepy, less alert, more forgetful, and overall less focused.

But officer, I only took fourteen pills! The doctor didn't tell me I would forget the speed limit!

We tend to minimize the dampening effect of this type of medication, since often patients will tell me that they feel fully alert and confident about their abilities, even after taking potent sedatives. Many of them find the calming effects highly seductive. In my view, and in the results of many research studies, most individuals on sedatives actually perform less effectively in many situations. Most patients evaluated by a neuropsychologist (a specialized psychologist trained to measure and assess how the brain is working) would clearly struggle with many areas of cognitive functioning. For many patients, the trade-off is justified, especially if their high level of anxiety interferes with their quality of life or ability to focus. One patient explained to me that she felt overwhelmed by the number of backed-up tax returns, unpaid bills, and collection notices piled on her desk. This sense of drowning in problems led her to a state of inertia and paralysis, which of course compounded her anxiety. Only when she had had a few cocktails was she able to pick up a few documents and start to chip away at the mountain of unopened mail and ominous notices from the IRS. (Not that the influence of alcohol would help most of us when we attempt to decipher the complex and convoluted instructions on the average 1040 form.)

Why can't I keep a little bottle in the office, like in the old days?

For others, such as surgeons, pilots, high-speed equities traders, or even that elderly man in the lane next to you on the freeway, the use of such inhibitory agents is far from ideal. You might speculate that, since we tend to utilize only 3 percent of our brain in our average day, taking away another half a percent would not be highly significant. But in reality, many of us are suffering significant impairments because of our medication regimens. Just because these substances do not show up on a Breathalyzer or are not classified as street drugs does not vindicate them as benign in everyday life. This becomes a difficult decision for us prescribing physicians. Just how much mood stabilizing medication is necessary to prevent a setback for our bipolar patient? We know that lithium, Depakote, and other similar agents will have some negative impact on our patients' ability to focus effectively. So how do we weigh the risk of a manic episode versus limiting someone's ability to succeed at work, school, or home?

Our colleagues in neurology face a similar dilemma, but in view of their goal of preventing a seizure, which is a highly dramatic and potentially life-threatening event, the use of high doses of three or four agents is not uncommon. I am often startled by some of these drug regimens but generally have noted very little resistance on the part of their patients. When it comes to a mood disorder, on the other hand, most of my patients, as well as their families and society as a whole, have very little tolerance for side effects. "I won't take it if I end up gaining even an ounce." "If it makes me tired, I will flush it down the toilet." "I just don't feel right on that medication, Doc." These are all protests that I have fielded over the years from a variety of disgruntled individuals. They all share a common reluctance to endure any adverse reactions, however unlikely or trivial in nature.

Why do we need serotonin, anyway?

Here things get even more complicated. We initially viewed serotonin as a substance that was protective, to some extent, against suicidal or violent behavior. This led to the development of Prozac, which of course emerged as a well-tolerated treatment for depressive disorders. In the course of becoming familiar with the treatment process, clinicians observed that most patients on Prozac also experienced a much lower level of anxiety, especially since about 70 percent of depressed patients also have a coexisting anxiety disorder. In the past twenty years, this class of medications—selective serotonin reuptake inhibitors—has been utilized primarily for a variety of anxiety disorders.

Against this clinical backdrop, scientists then studied the areas of the brain that appeared to rely mainly on serotonin transmission. These areas tended to become activated when the individual experienced fear or alarm. The purpose of serotonin, from an adaptive perspective, is thus related to alerting the subject to potential danger. Reducing the intensity of serotonin-based activity became an effective method of mitigating the sense of anxiety or tension that anxious patients suffer from, even in nonthreatening situations.

But what if it feels like I'm having a heart attack?

Here again it is helpful to look at the biological basis for behavior. Over the past ten thousand years, as our brains became more and more fine-tuned and developed, we followed Darwin's basic principle of evolution—only the fittest survive. So those Homo sapiens who didn't check their cave for a grizzly bear or failed to stock up enough berries and nuts to make it through a long, harsh winter, did not live long enough to pass on their genes. The world was in fact quite a dangerous and hostile place. So the role of fear and alarm centers in the brain was quite essential.

Modern-day humankind has to face threats of a different nature, but, for most of us, these are not life or death matters. Being called into the boss's office should not trigger a fight-or-flight response, but, given the economy these days and the unreasonable supervisors out there, perhaps it should. Having a rude driver cut you off should not cause your adrenal glands to pump out massive amounts of adrenaline, leading to the condition we refer to as road rage, but it often does. Having an argument with one's partner about whose family to spend Christmas day with is not likely to lead to any harm to life or limb, but many of us would rather consider sacrificing a limb rather than facing this conflict. From these commonplace examples, you can see that we are programmed to respond in a fairly dramatic fashion when we perceive some sort of danger. Unfortunately, that danger can be as benign as an elevator or supermarket for many of my patients.

What if I don't have time to let the Prozac kick in?

Here we note that most of our widely used medications that revolve around the chemical serotonin have two major drawbacks—they may take three to six weeks for maximum impact, and they often make the person's anxiety even more unpleasant in the first week of treatment. So the next step for the pharmaceutical companies involved coming up with a reliable method of reducing a patient's level of distress on a short-term or immediate basis. This class of medications—the sedatives—relies, as I have discussed, on a chemical called GABA, the primary inhibitory chemical in the brain. This means that any agent that enhances GABA transmission will help calm activity in the brain, whether triggered or spontaneous.

As noted above, damping down the brain's level of activity has some definite downsides. Most of us want our brains to function at maximum capacity, so we logically would avoid any agent that impedes the chemical and electrical processes that allow us to think and feel. On the other hand, when we are suffering from a severe seizure or a miserable panic attack, dampening the level of distress by whatever means is desirable.

How do I stay focused and alert when I feel like taking a siesta?

This takes us back to the time when we believed that the vast majority of mood and anxiety disorders were mediated by norepinephrine, a stimulating chemical produced by the brain but also the adrenal gland. This chemical helps us remain alert, focused, and productive, though an excess of this, also known as norepi, can lead to panic attacks or even a form of catatonia.

What's the most fun-loving neurotransmitter?

Of these chemicals, the one that most of us would prefer for short- or long-term use would be dopamine. This is the life of the party:

it helps us get motivated, appreciate social and recreational events, enjoy social interactions, and keep moving in general. Dopamine is not only helpful for energy and cognitive focus, but it also helps to power the "reward center" in the brain. Though many of us speak of having a "runner's high" that results from the secretion of endorphins, our natural opioids, most of us are not likely to experience this level of gratification. The average American is not likely to partake in an extended exercise outing of at least fifty minutes, which is necessary to raise one's endorphin levels. We are instead likely to benefit from the much more immediate secretion of an important neurotransmitter called dopamine, which can spike in our blood stream just seconds into a positive and intense social, vocational, or recreational experience. Medications that raise one's dopamine level in a potent manner thus tend to be highly addictive. This might include cocaine, amphetamines, and other stimulants.

What about too much of a good thing?

One might wonder why the pharmaceutical industry can't come up with a long-acting dopamine-enhancing agent that we could all take advantage of. Where's the downside of a chemical that is found naturally in the brain and that miraculously makes us happy, motivated, focused, and energized? Here we have to consider the impact of dopamine when taken to the nth degree. In clinical experience, we observe that those patients who abuse large doses of amphetamines or cocaine tend to develop a severe and treatment-resistant paranoid psychosis, rather than a sense of well-being. In fact, the most paranoid individual I have ever treated entered the hospital with the terrifying conviction that the Terminator was hunting her down and in fact was likely to squeeze through the keyhole of the psychiatric unit where she was admitted. It was only after five days of intensive therapy with dopamine-blocking agents that she finally realized that her fears were based on a Hollywood blockbuster and were not based in reality.

The second concern, of course, would be addiction. If a modest amount of dopamine makes you happy, then why not double your pleasure and take twice the dose? This also relates to the brain's tendency to become tolerant of a chemical process, to the point that we need a higher dosage to attain the same clinical effect.

On a positive note, we do have some lower-potency agents that do enhance dopamine transmission and only rarely are associated with psychosis, addiction, or tolerance. These include an antidepressant called Wellbutrin, which has been out on the market since 1989, and the highly potent group of antidepressants that you might have read about as having a severe and dangerous reaction with a variety of over-the-counter cold preparations. These are the MAO inhibitors, which are effective in many cases of treatment-resistant mood disorders. This class has a powerful broad-spectrum impact on not just one or two but three critical chemicals that regulate mood and anxiety. Unfortunately they tend to be neglected due to potentially severe interactions with certain foods and medications. In my experience a motivated patient who is reliable and focuses reasonably well deserves the opportunity to undergo MAOI treatment prior to being referred for electroconvulsive therapy.

How do we explain all those smokers and coffee fiends out there?

Here we have the opportunity to discuss the most commonly used mind-altering substances (also known as psychotropics) in the world. This dynamic and lucrative duo includes caffeine and nicotine. Both help to generate huge sums of money and demand much of our time and energy. How many everyday products would we spend nine dollars a day on? How many beans would we take the time to purchase, grind, percolate, and then modify with various sweeteners, creams, and other additives?

So, starting with the Starbucks phenomenon, let's focus on caffeine. How does caffeine affect the brain to the point that PepsiCo, Coca-Cola, and Starbucks have all become massive international enterprises? These products have a less potent effect than the prescription stimulants, but they have a consistent and noticeable impact on our functional status and mood nonetheless. While many of us are more willing to pay large sums in search of relaxation, the vast majority tend to be frustrated by their perceived lack of energy, focus, and motivation. Anyone who is able to obtain a reasonable dose of caffeine, which of course tends to be served in convenient drive-throughs these days, has the ability to modify their energy levels and focus, albeit for a short time. Out of all my inpatients and outpatients over the past twenty-two years, I cannot consider more than 5 percent of them as complaining of having too much energy. The vast majority of us are generally seeking any edge which might help us get through the day in a more focused and efficient manner.

As for nicotine, this is quite a fascinating agent. As any smoker will happily reveal, if he or she is overly tense, a dose of nicotine seems to relieve this state. If he or she is instead fatigued and struggling to stay focused, a cigarette can help with remaining alert and addressing tasks more efficiently. This is quite difficult to compete with, of course, so often encouraging one of my patients to quit can feel like a lost cause. Nicotine can in fact maximize your ability to retain information. So, even though we nonsmokers might groan in dismay, smokers may actually have an advantage when it comes to forming memories. This often justifies the decision to prolong a patient's use of nicotine, which, to my knowledge, is quite benign in the absence of tar and other toxins which lurk in the cloud of cigarette or cigar smoke.

Chapter 6

Basic Pharmacology Made Simple

Just as every field boasts a complex jargon, which is expressly utilized to keep the rest of us in utter confusion, my field has many terms and specific medications. We have hundreds of self-professed or widely promoted experts who glibly speak of serotonin, rejection sensitivity, and REM sleep deprivation. Our treatment options are not nearly as complicated, however, as the underlying triggers for the disorders that we target. Our field fortunately offers only four major types of medications, which generally appear self-explanatory, but unfortunately can be quite confusing in actual practice:

1) Antidepressants

2) Mood stabilizers

3) Antipsychotics

4) Sedatives

Antidepressants, or "Doc, I just need a happy pill"

Back in the roaring '90s, when I started my training, the field of psychiatry was thrilled by the sight of a shiny new capsule on the cover of *Time* magazine. This was Prozac, the revolutionary antidepressant that many of my colleagues have argued should be universally prescribed. One of my fellow residents advocated adding Prozac to the water supply. This agent has been promoted for dozens of uses and has been featured in many books, articles, and condemnations. But this blockbuster preparation, the first of the SSRIs (or serotonin reuptake inhibitors), was only the first of a growing pack of antidepressants. The confusion ensues when we start to discuss individual agents. "Why did that doctor pick Zoloft rather than Effexor?" "Why didn't he pick the one with that great commercial—the one with the dog holding the leash in his mouth and waiting by the door?"

Mood Stabilizers or "What goes up must come down"

When the market for depressive patients and the so-called worried well became saturated, we had the bipolar craze in the second half of the '90s. Suddenly everyone who racked up a big credit card bill at Macy's, yelled at their spouse, or drove too fast on the freeway was no longer just making poor decisions; they were bipolar. Naturally we all like to explain our irrational behavior in some sort of rational fashion, and this is where the field of psychiatry has often bailed us out. This led to a boom, not for the traditional (and inexpensive) proven therapies for mood swings, including lithium and some long-acting sedatives such as Klonopin, but instead for a new generation of antiseizure agents. Many of these medications, which we borrowed from our neurology colleagues, were found to have a measurable benefit for those of us who truly fall into the category formerly known as manic depression. These patients in fact develop true manic episodes, which often do respond to mood stabilizers, though only a select few have been clinically proven. We have some legitimate offerings here, including Depakote and Lamictal, as well as some wannabees that didn't pan out in clinical trials, such as Topamax, Neurontin, and Trileptal. Many of these agents are also used for impulse control disorders, though in my experience they do not generally prevent my patients or neighbors from spending excessively or verbally abusing the umpire who calls his son out at the plate. On the other hand, in past studies (that would not be allowed today due to ethical concerns), prisoners were given lithium, in spite of lacking a formal psychiatric diagnosis. This in fact led to a marked reduction in the frequency of fighting or violence in these prisons, which supported a role for lithium in helping control impulses with or without an actual diagnosis of bipolar disorder. Please don't give this to your teenagers when they act up, however, unless an adolescent psychiatrist or behavioral pediatrician gives the green light!

Antipsychotics or "Whatever happened to Thorazine?"

In the past decade, once we had exhausted the potential for adding mood stabilizers to our patients' regimens with any hint of mood swings or "cycling," we ushered in a new generation of tranquilizers—the so-called atypical agents. Who hasn't seen commercials for these agents, with a serious moderator asking you to speak with your doctor about a possible diagnosis of bipolar and to consider a trial of Abilify or Seroquel? Unfortunately, these agents are best at doing two things, as you can surmise from their names. First, they will tranquilize you, with both a reduced level of anxiety and lessened mental and physical activity. Second, given additional time, usually up to two or three weeks, they will generally eliminate or at least markedly diminish any psychotic thoughts or behaviors. Any other use could clearly be questioned and often has been, by many critical practitioners, agencies, and concerned public groups. While there is clearly a role for these agents, at times one could argue that their use is akin to using a revolver to kill a mosquito. They will get the job done, but there might be some serious collateral damage.

If at first you don't succeed, try, try again!

The next incarnation of these agents emerged just as the market for bipolar patients, who by this time were running for the hills, became overly crowded and competitive. This was in fact the holy grail of the field—treating those patients who just don't seem to get better. Most patients whom I have had the good fortune to evaluate and treat have had past trials of various medications and have sought input from their relatives, friends, and usually their primary care or other non-psychiatrist physicians. Their condition is thus likely to fall into the category of a treatment-resistant mood disorder, having had at least two comprehensive but unsuccessful trials of antidepressant therapy. This is where the field can become more treacherous, with dozens of partially effective options but precious few with real, clinically proven efficacy. Even the medications that we read about in magazines or that we see in high-tech commercials have limited benefit compared to placebos. In defense of my misunderstood specialty, I would argue that all medical fields have their challenges, in which many patients improve but only to a limited extent. This includes victims of strokes, congestive heart failure, dementia, etc. We thus are generally satisfied with any options that might lead to a greater than 50 percent response.

We have used tranquilizers in this capacity for several decades for a variety of mood and anxiety disorders. When added to an antidepressant, many antipsychotic agents have been helpful in either elevating a depressed mood or stabilizing a volatile one. Of course, there are few dramatic cures, but in conjunction with a solid therapy program, a reasonable support system, and a chance to garner some small successes, a patient with chronic depression has every likelihood of getting better. Perhaps only 5 to 10 percent will have a minimal response, which in my book is pretty good odds.

Sedatives, or "20 20 24 hours a day, I want to be sedated" (with apologies to the talented Ramones)

The last group of agents is the most popular, by a long shot. Over the past few thousand years, this has included herbal agents, such as Valerian root; opioids such as laudanum and opium; barbiturates such as Seconal; a new generation of agents called benzodiazepines, including Valium, Xanax, Librium, Klonopin, etc.; and a related class of sleeping agents including Lunesta, Ambien, and Sonata. Their huge popularity clearly results from their ability to address fairly rapidly most symptoms of anxiety, insomnia, and agitation. These sedatives, also known as minor tranquillizers, are the cleanest of the bunch in many respects. They have few effects other than sedating us. They don't cause weight gain, tremors, diabetes, or erectile dysfunction (unless they make us fall asleep). This has led to many millions of Valium prescriptions, and more recently has shifted to the use of Xanax, which is lamentably our number one requested—and prescribed—agent.

The original sedative was of course fermented and consumed thousands of years ago. Alcohol was invented several millennia ago and has been co-opted into serving a myriad of purposes, which naturally include "taking the edge off" (or reducing) anxiety. Of course, alcohol is quite curious in the sense that many imbibers become more, rather than less, animated. This wonderful substance has many positive properties, including the following:

1) Taking away our inhibitions and thus allowing us to enjoy interactions and events more fully

2) Helping provide more energy when we are fatigued

3) Helping us sleep when we are overly tense

4) Helping relax our muscles when they are tight

5) Helping us deal with emotional pain when we are overwhelmed (Think of the Irish funeral.)

6) Enhancing our mood when we are having fun, and convincing us we are having fun even when we may not be

Of course there is no free lunch. The potential drawbacks of alcohol seem to be a dirty little secret, both to our patients who want a quick fix that they can carry in their pocketbooks and take as needed, and to us clinicians as well. As a result of pressures on the practice of my specialty and medicine in general, psychiatrists unfortunately seem to be relying more and more on Band-Aid pharmaceutical solutions, rather than taking the time and energy to work through a difficult situation or emotion with a patient. Some potential drawbacks of using sedatives include the following:

1) Impaired memory and concentration. Perhaps we tend to forget how lousy we have been feeling.

2) Impaired motor coordination. This does not help with operating cars or drill presses.

3) Reduced effectiveness over time—a phenomenon labeled tolerance. This leads to the necessity for a gradual increase in the dosage of these agents with time.

4) Severe and potentially lethal interactions with other sedatives or narcotics, including alcohol, painkillers, and sleeping medication.

5) As noted above in the addiction section, about 15 percent of patients will develop problematic use of these agents, with a variety of complications.

6) Lastly, these agents interfere with one's ability to cope with stress in the long run. They do not allow the patient to learn new techniques to manage adversity but instead serve as a means of sweeping problems under the rug. At times they have even been implicated in triggering or exacerbating a depressive episode.

Patients tend to roll their eyes when I run through this list, unless they have personally experienced one or more of these setbacks themselves in the past. Often by the time they arrive at my office, they have exhausted such treatments offered by other clinicians: "Xanax was great in the beginning, but it just doesn't last that long anymore." "Recently I have to take two Ambiens to fall asleep." "I can only take half a Klonopin or my boss starts to ask me if I'm okay." The initial promise of these agents is quite powerful, however, and difficult to resist when we are in distress. Plus, we are to a large extent conditioned by the media and the pharmaceutical industry to think that any problem can be addressed overnight, provided that you are willing to "talk with your doctor."

Why should we worry about these potential side effects? As most of my patients state with conviction, "It won't happen to me." And "Xanax is the only thing that helps, Doc." Back in the '70s, it was Valium that prompted many office visits, though for some reason this agent has virtually vanished. But the same issues and baggage that tainted Valium's image over the years accompany the use of any of these sister agents.

Then again, I have always been curious about the fact that many patients tell me that Xanax cures their panic attack in a matter of minutes, though the time required to absorb and distribute a medication might appear incompatible with their experience. This leads to my understanding of this process in which the patient's anxiety subsides just by virtue of the act of having swallowed a pill. They are convinced of this phenomenon, even though there is no measurable level of this agent in one's blood until long after the panic attack has resolved. This leads to our next topic: the power of positive or even wishful thinking.

The Wonderful Placebo Effect

We know that the vast majority of patients improve substantially, even if we just spend some time, offer them a comfortable guest chair, and offer them a placebo. This has been proven repeatedly, to the distress of many specialists who take offense at the fact that whichever wonderful plan they concoct will demonstrate limited superiority over a simple diagnostic session complete with a sugar pill. This effect has at times led large-scale studies to challenge many long-established medical and psychiatric treatments. We find that the difference between our active treatment plan and the dummy treatment is in fact quite limited. For example, a given antidepressant might help 74 percent of a given population, while a placebo somehow helped almost 50 percent. So in this case, only 24 percent truly responded to the pharmaceutical product. Rather than taking it personally, I embrace this phenomenon. Why not get a running start? This means that, even if I fail to choose the optimal treatment, the odds are still in my favor.

While this effect can be quite confusing, after twenty-one years of clinical experience, I have come to a reasonable understanding of it. I know that when I choose to consult another doctor for my own benefit, I find myself feeling much improved before I even leave his or her office. From my perspective, just learning that I have a condition that is treatable and is not going to kill me or cause any of my parts to atrophy and fall off is worth every penny of that dreaded copayment.

How do you pick a medication—there are so many out there!

This is always a major concern when I start a relatively new patient on any medication. I have had initial sessions where I tried to squeeze eight months of intensive pharmacology lectures into fifty-five minutes. If you think that's easy, try reading *War and Peace* in a weekend. Patients have so many different sources for information and often surprise me with new reasons for choosing a particular medication. It mostly comes down to the same criteria that people use to pick a plumber or a brand of dishwasher—word of mouth. "My neighbor did great on Lexapro; he's like a new man." "My mother-in-law is a barrel of monkeys ever since she started on Zoloft." It's hard to argue with direct personal experience. So often I take advantage of someone's interest to get a running start. If someone believes in a product, for whatever nonscientific reason, that's good enough for me. (See above, discussion about the placebo effect.) But when a patient gives me carte blanche to make a recommendation (which rarely happens), what is my selection process? Good question, and one that is answered by examining the following flow chart:

Seven Steps in Selecting a Medication Regimen

1) Establish diagnosis, and choose medications that ideally are FDA-approved for that diagnosis. Does the given medication have a research-based FDA indication for the problem or diagnosis that we are trying to address?
2) Explore the patient's tolerance of side effects, and minimize risk of undesired adverse effects. Does the medication commonly lead to any side effects that the patient is absolutely unwilling to tolerate?
3) Explore family history, which may reveal an agent that has helped a close relative. Does the patient have any first-degree relatives who have had a promising response to a specific agent?
4) Discuss financial and/or insurance limitations, and choose cost-effective treatments as much as possible. Does the patient have any specific financial limitations that would argue for a generic product?
5) Establish the patient's preference for standing vs. as- needed medications, and proceed accordingly when possible. Does the patient prefer a regularly administered agent or rather one that he or she would take as needed?

6) Elicit any history of addiction and choose non-addictive medications when possible.

7) Discuss any co-existing conditions and formulate a plan with the simplest possible medication regimen. Is there a medication that might help with more than one of the patient's clinical issues? For example, most patients with mood issues suffer from anxiety as well. As noted above, most antidepressants in the serotonin-based family will address both mood and anxiety disorders. Another antidepressant has been approved for smoking cessation, so I may prescribe it for a patient who is trying to quit smoking, in addition to needing a mood elevator. Naturally as a physician who is highly concerned with my patients' overall health, I am overjoyed to assist a smoker with this goal. Other medications appear to be helpful for ADD patients, though this effect is not as potent as that of amphetamines.

In general I inform patients that the first priority is stabilizing their mood. After that, other problems can be identified, targeted, and managed.

Doctor Pete, I feel like a guinea pig!

This relates to point number one from the above list. In fact, virtually all medication regimens that I propose to my outpatients are based on well-established research studies on large numbers of real-world patients. I always inform my patients that, once we are confident about their diagnostic picture, we have a solid basis for intervening with a targeted and scientific treatment. When I see new patients who hand me laundry lists of medical and psychiatric medications, most of which they do not recognize or appreciate, I often find myself frustrated. Each medication has to pull its own weight and be appropriate for the specific condition for which it is intended. Then each disorder must be periodically reevaluated in order to ascertain whether the treatment program warrants any fine-tuning or other adjustment. Simply deciding to add additional agents or blindly increasing dosages is not a valid game plan, but sadly it is common practice. The initial interview in my office often results in a reduction— rather than increase—in medication. This often catches new patients off guard. Once they understand that less is usually more when it comes to effective treatment, and that any dead weight is better off being shed, they appreciate my methods. Any medication that is not clearly helping my patient get better or stay better ends up on the chopping block. When, on occasion, sacrificing a medication leads to a clinical setback, we are generally able to regroup and restart therapy with that medication, which has then proven its value. Of course this process is much simpler when a patient or his family is able to present a clear history. This would provide a reasonable review of treatment over an appropriate time frame, including onset of treatment, subsequent medication changes, and benefits, side effects, and other relevant data.

Speaking of side effects brings us to point number two. Here we must clearly determine which potential side effects a patient is entirely unwilling to entertain. For example, a young bride with anxiety about intimacy with her persistent husband would be unlikely to continue on any medication that had a dampening effect on her libido. The majority of commuters, who battle morning traffic long before I am even capable of perusing the *New York Times*, would be loath to consider taking a medication that leads to severe grogginess or sedation in the morning. Any patient with a tendency to gain weight would tend to dismiss any medication that would feed this insidious trend. So this discussion needs to occur on day one.

To be perfectly honest, this concern appears somewhat exaggerated to my eye in the sense that any medication that leads to undesirable effects can be summarily stopped, metabolized, and promptly cleared from one's system. Most patients would clearly prefer to avoid this process, however, and are quick to question me about the exhaustive list of possible side effects that the pharmacist, the PDR, the Internet, or their second cousin twice removed provided for them.

What about those scary warnings that you see on TV commercials?

This is a major controversy that has complicated my work immensely. In its infinite wisdom, our federal government has decided to convey warnings of both common and rare side effects with no indication of frequency. In other words, patients are faced with a laundry list of potential side effects, from mild dizziness to death, with little perspective on what to expect in the real world. We all know that in extremely rare cases any given medication can trigger an allergy, which in extreme cases can result in what we call an anaphylactic response. This includes respiratory distress and can lead to death. Other rare reactions might include Stevens-Johnson syndrome, in which one's skin becomes inflamed and sloughs off. This can lead to admission to a burn unit and at times can be fatal. Have I seen these complications in twenty-two years of practice? Not yet. I hope to retire in another twenty-two years in the same blissful ignorance of these frightening conditions.

Can the medication make me worse?

This is an interesting phenomenon that does have some clinical basis. During my training, I was taught to monitor a patient who presents with severe depressive features quite closely. The concern is that an individual who has ongoing hopelessness and suicidal thoughts might be too incapacitated to act on these thoughts. As he or she undergoes the initial phases of treatment and gains more energy and motivation, the risk of suicidal behavior might increase rather than decline. So when I start an acutely ill patient on a new regimen I ask them (and their families) to update me about any possible setbacks. I frequently check my office for calls. I inform them that their symptoms might worsen in the short term rather than improve. Should I feel that the risk of self-injurious behavior is high, I refer them to a safe setting such as an inpatient unit. Lastly, I check on the patient often, by making periodic phone calls as well as by setting up regular office visits. So this should all make sense to you as common sense practice.

On a related note, a common question from patients and their families has resulted from the government's decision to issues a strong warning about the following rare but serious adverse reaction. A small percentage of patients who are started on mood-elevating or stabilizing agents appear to experience a higher level of suicidal thoughts. This appears to constitute about two percent or less of given patients, but is startling nonetheless. Fortunately, there is no connection between having these thoughts and actually acting on them. My understanding is that a patient who is severely withdrawn or fatigued might start to express preexisting feelings as he or she starts to respond to treatment. In other words, the individual might have had the same hopelessness prior to initiating treatment but were not able or willing to impart this to his or her family or to the treatment team. I cannot confirm this theory and would certainly have difficulty designing a study to prove its accuracy, but I make this claim based on more than two decades of clinical experience. In addition, many well-conducted studies have demonstrated that a large percentage of patients who are considering suicide do not share this with their families or doctors. Regrettably, many patients who in fact attempt or complete suicide have seen a health care provider in the month prior to their suicide attempt. This might argue for the possibility that a patient who has started treatment might be more likely to have increased contact with his or her treatment team, which might lead the individual to divulge more of his or her inner thoughts and feelings.

The current message that the FDA has required is that any given agent for mood disorders must be accompanied by the warning that the patient might experience increased suicidal thoughts. The vast majority of my colleagues and I fear that this well-intentioned warning may have prevented thousands of patients from seeking or following through with potentially life-saving treatment. In fact, since these warnings have been widely publicized, several studies have demonstrated an increased rate of suicide in adolescents, a group in which this risk was felt to be higher. Ultimately the warning clearly may have led to more harm than good, though, as they say, you can't fight City Hall.

What if my whole family is taking Prozac?

When I learn that a patient has a strong family history of a certain disorder, of course my ears perk up. This is not only helpful in pinning down a diagnosis but also helps me immensely with choosing a course of action. If a patient tells me that her brother has responded extremely well to cognitive therapy, it would be silly to rely exclusively on medications. If someone tells me that his grandfather was a mean son of a gun until he started taking Paxil at the age of ninety-two, I will definitely file that information away. If the patient's mother tells me she's been taking lithium for the past thirty years, that also can be relevant. By the same token, if someone tells me that everyone in the family is taking Valium, that might trigger my clinical radar. If the family history includes suicidal behavior, then I really have to be vigilant.

But Doc, my pharmacy bill is like another mortgage payment!

The fourth area revolves around the plain reality that many folks lack access to treatment based on economic barriers. Many times over the course of my career, starting in Spanish Harlem, to the Bronx, and then to the Jersey Shore, I have heard that a medication has been helpful but is not affordable. Many patients thus take their chances and wean off a medication that had demonstrated dramatic improvements in their quality of life and functionality. This always rubs me the wrong way, in that the wealthiest country in the world should not ask its citizens to choose between paying the rent, feeding the children, and taking medications that can be transformative. Fortunately there are many solutions for this perennial landmine. We no longer have the luxury of asking the cash-strapped pharmacies to donate medication for indigent patients but instead have to appeal to the good will of the pharmaceutical companies. Whether their good will derives from the need for public relations, tax write-offs, or simply ethical principles and corporate generosity, these companies simply give away vast amounts of medication each year. This could be in the form of free coupons, samples at hospitals or clinics, or even personal supplies that are mailed to my office for distribution or directly to the needy patient's home. Unfortunately many patients just assume that their medications are out of reach. So here I have an opportunity to educate and to serve as a caseworker. Despite the existence of these support programs, I currently have several patients who are purchasing medication on the Internet, from India, or from friends or family who may have superior prescription plans.

Why can't I just take something when I need it?

I always encounter patients who have a clear-cut aversion to taking medications on a regular schedule. They tell me in a convincing manner that they are generally successful in managing their anxiety and that their mood tends to be quite upbeat. For this reason they prefer to forgo any daily dosing schedule, and they usually request a supply of some sedative that they can carry from place to place in the event of an anxiety attack. For the most part, this plan is clearly not ideal, as I pointed out in my earlier discussion about sedatives that are generally employed in such a situational approach. I tend to offer my own preference, which coincides with the saying that "an ounce of prevention is worth a pound of cure." Many studies have proven that, just as a patient in physical distress will ultimately use a higher dose of analgesics for relief if he has to wait until his pain becomes severe, a patient with a severe anxiety disorder will tend to require a higher dose of sedative if he waits until his anxiety escalates into a panic attack. For better or for worse, many patients also prefer immediate measures that will take effect in twenty or thirty minutes, rather than three or four weeks. We are exposed to many messages as we come of age, most of which promise a (commercially generated) solution for virtually any difficulty. We also are raised to expect an immediate result and do not tolerate delayed gratification very well. This leads to considerable frustration when I attempt to explain to my outpatients the rationale for withholding short-acting medications. This frustration may even extend to my patients' long-suffering families, who also object to my hard-nosed stance. Here is a recent e-mail from one of my so-called bipolar patient's parents:

Hi doctor,

Sorry to bother you but we need some help. Since her med change, she [his twenty-seven-year-old daughter] has been very uptight, irritable, arguing, and fighting with everyone. She was so frustrated the other day that she said that she should be in a padded room with a punching bag. Or even that she could "strangle someone." When we try to calm her down, she gets mad and says, "You all know how to push my buttons!"

Is it possible that she could be put on Xanax again or some other medicine?

In this case I certainly feel like the bad guy. Why take away a sedative that appears to soothe the anger of an angry patient? This not only leads to a negative outcome for her family, but also to feelings of guilt and remorse on her part. So why would her doctor withhold something that might help her "calm down?"

Well, for one, as I noted in the section on sedatives, these medications can lead to amnesia. If we rely on a sedative in any circumstance in which we feel angry or overwhelmed, this will ultimately impair our ability to tolerate or manage these challenging situations. Having recourse to a martini or a sedative engenders a form of escapism, which in the long term tends to perpetuate these episodes of anger or other forms of lack of control.

The second concern is that the patient is not facing the consequences of her hostile or otherwise inappropriate actions. She is no longer accountable for her behavior but instead is given the message that acting out behavior will be addressed with a sedative. In the end such a response does not help someone learn to control his or her actions. In the case of the twenty-seven-year old woman, I responded that the preferable approach—aside from making use of a mood stabilizer that would ideally help moderate the patient's impulsive behavior—would be to draw up a clear and consistent behavioral plan. This either written or verbal contract would help the patient recognize that any aggressive or hostile behavior would lead either to immediate disengagement or eventually to some other form of negative reinforcement. Though it can take considerable time for a twenty-seven year old to modify her patterns of engagement with her family and/or peers, this is the only definitive means of making headway. The critical point is that it will take a concerted effort for the family to modify their own patterns and reactions in order to facilitate this process. To presume that we can say or do something to "calm someone down" is quite unrealistic, as far as I am concerned, for two major reasons:

1) It is difficult enough to modify our own behavior. To control someone else's behavior is utterly impossible.

2) Every patient in my practice—aside from those who are grossly psychotic and out of touch with reality—is accountable for his or her own behavior and well-being. If we attempt to appease an angry patient or subdue them with sedatives, we are violating this principle and in fact enabling their hostile and maladaptive behavior.

These behavioral contracts do not lead to much excitement when presented to my patients and their families. In fact, the basic principles and guidelines tend to strike most of them as obvious and commonplace. In the heat of the moment, however, many of these basic concepts fly out the window. Here is an example of a contract that might be helpful in this context:

1) If I am angry, I can express this in several ways, such as keeping a journal, telling a friend or family member about it in a calm manner, or speaking with my therapist when he or she is available.

2) If I speak in an abusive or hostile manner to others, they will point this out once. If this is not successful in helping me regain control, they will leave the premises and ask me to find another means of expressing myself.

3) If I start to become threatening or pose a potential danger in any way, my family or friends have the right to call for an intervention, even if I am not in agreement.

4) If I fail to focus on my treatment in a healthy manner, my family or friends have the right to include themselves in this process to help with my recovery.

Why take away something that works?

Most of those anxious folks who find themselves relying on sedatives are unable to achieve a state of relaxation, even with the addition of a primary medication such as an antidepressant, which theoretically will take over for the short-term agent. In clinical experience, however, about 15 percent of patients exposed to short- or long-term use of sedatives are at risk of becoming addicted to these medications. This of course can take the form of either a physical or psychological dependence, but usually is based on the latter when dealing with a depressed or anxious client. These patients find it quite tempting to take a regular dose of Xanax to "take the edge off" but eventually start to crave a more frequent or higher dose. At times they end up revealing this trend to me, though some of them become fearful of repercussions and will invent stories in order to obtain a larger supply of medication. Others will find additional prescribers to avoid a shortfall. Naturally these folks are highly prone to the plethora of complications noted above in the discussion about sedatives.

How do we take care of more than one problem?

In many cases patients expect me to come up with a simple treatment program for a complex set of issues. This can be quite difficult, as you might imagine. On the other hand, many medications that modulate or help regulate one's serotonin metabolism can address a variety of anxiety disorders as well as mood disorders. This does simplify my work, in that about 70 percent of patients with mood disorders also have anxiety issues. So, starting any given patient on Paxil or a similar medication can provide several benefits. Any patient with panic attacks, generalized anxiety disorder, OCD, or even posttraumatic disorder has a high likelihood of benefiting from Paxil. This will help obviate the need for several medications, as long as each one is carefully chosen and ends up carrying its weight. This process can be extremely satisfying when I am on occasion able to hit the nail on the head in order to alleviate a patient's panic attacks as well as obsessive compulsive behavior and a coexisting depressive syndrome.

The more the merrier—except when it comes to pharmaceuticals.

Unfortunately what commonly occurs over an extended period of time is that, while we initially started a number of medications in a considered, rational fashion, with time this process can become somewhat haphazard. We might be reluctant to jeopardize a new patient's stability by weaning them off of existing medications. In many cases, we thus find ourselves adding more medications when we note that the patient has had only a partial or limited response. Most of us are reluctant to take away something that might potentially be helpful, lest an already struggling patient might deteriorate even more. So the pattern unfortunately becomes a series of add-ons to an often complex multitude of medications, which of course increases the likelihood of adverse reactions and cost to the patient and the health care system.

Often when I ask patients which medications are helpful, or even what each one is designed to address, they shrug their shoulders and ask me to call their prior treating clinicians. This can result in some extensive detective work that would keep Sherlock Holmes busy for a month. In a perfect world, patients would walk into my office with a detailed list in chronological order, starting with their first medication trial and extending up to the present. Each phase of treatment would be described, including targeted symptoms, clinical response, any adverse effects or allergies, and reasons for stopping, if applicable. This would certainly facilitate my work of choosing a new regimen, though, to be fair, with some prompting on my part, most of my patients are able to provide a reasonable history. While naturally any prior psychiatrists who are available to provide their perspective would be invaluable, this exchange of information does not always take place. In the real world, which entails time pressure and ever decreasing reimbursement, many of us find that the time necessary to become fully acquainted with a new client is no longer compensated in a fair manner, and we start to take shortcuts. While I would be the last to support such a trend, I do recognize that my colleagues, who have devoted much of their youth to pursuing a medical degree, are entitled to a reasonable quality of life in their everyday work.

What about if I somehow benefit from a side effect?

This is an interesting perspective. From my vantage point it can be quite helpful to make use of adverse effects of a medication, since many of these can work in your favor. In fact, many of our older medications were designed to have another therapeutic action, which was superseded by the novel psychotropic activity. For example, Thorazine, a well-known tranquilizer and antipsychotic, started out as an antihistamine. In modern day psychiatry very few patients are maintained on this complicated and at times hazardous drug, but those of us who actually desire some sedation or relief from a case of allergic rhinitis (a.k.a. hay fever) might be quite satisfied. Those of us who have lost excessive weight for a variety of reasons—primarily due to severe anxiety and tension—would clearly benefit from many of my favorite medications' tendency to restore the appetite, not only by relieving the patient's anxiety but in addition through a direct effect on the hunger center in the brain. This could include many first-generation antidepressants as well as several new-generation tranquilizers, such as Zyprexa and Seroquel. When it comes to helping with weight loss, as my typical reader already knows, the range of options is much slimmer. We might offer a course of Topamax at times as a potential mood stabilizer, though this is not an FDA-approved indication. Or perhaps a healthy dose of Effexor, or even Prozac, for that matter, might help address certain cases of compulsive eating behavior and thereby lead to weight loss. Many older-generation medications were helpful in addressing anxiety and sleep disturbances due to intrinsic sedation, which often becomes a source of frustration after several weeks of struggling with drowsiness and the temptation to return to bed. Many newer medications have a number of sexual side effects, most commonly a slowing down of the sexual response. This can in fact be a useful phenomenon for a young patient who fears an overly rapid response and develops severe anxiety in this arena. Delayed ejaculation for some folks can be a blessing for others. The reduced libido that some patients develop can be distressing, but in some cases it can be desirable. And we all know that stimulants, ranging from caffeine to amphetamines, have a range of popular effects, aside from helping those with ADD focus more effectively. Who would complain about a medication that not only helps you be more productive but also raises your energy level, helps you lose weight, boosts your libido, lifts your mood (albeit only temporarily), and overall makes you feel more competent and confident? Sounds like a winner to me. In fact the FDA has become so concerned about the widespread use of this class of medication that it decided to issue a bulletin about the cardiac risks of stimulant use. The reality is that these agents are quite safe and have been studied extensively in elderly hospitalized patients and found to have minimal toxicity. Common sense would dictate that any patient with a recent heart attack, stroke, or uncontrolled hypertension would not a good candidate. But just because you're ninety-four years old with various chronic medical issues doesn't mean that you can't benefit from a dose of Adderall. When a high-risk patient develops severe depressive symptoms, including anorexia, then a few doses of stimulant can help to start clearing the disorder quite rapidly with little downside.

What about for addiction disorders?

Here we have some good news. Those of you struggling with addictions to alcohol, drugs, or even other behaviors such as gambling, overspending, etc. now have recourse to some biological tools. Even though making use of a twelve-step program is still statistically the most effective means of managing an addiction, the impact of some of these medical interventions can be dramatic at times. I try to keep expectations for these medications fairly modest, since the last thing I want is to dissuade the patient from following a program in addition to the medication regimen. However, these options can clearly supplement an effective outpatient regimen.

For those patients who abuse alcohol, we have the old-school approach of using Antabuse. This chemical blocks an enzyme that breaks down alcohol, leading to a high level of aldehyde in the blood. This then leads to flushing, headaches, and a general sense of misery. Of course, those patients who fail to take Antabuse regularly or who skip a few doses and then find that their window of opportunity is wide open, are less likely to respond to this fairly low-tech intervention. The newer approaches include both Campral, a lesser known medication that helps to reduce alcohol cravings, as well as naltrexone, aka Revia, a second drug that relieves cravings. In addition, when a patient relapses on Revia, they tend to consume much smaller quantities of alcohol.

The use of naltrexone has also been widespread in treating addictions to pain killers or opioids. This agent will effectively block any impact from the use of opioids. In addition, the fortunate patient also finds that his or her interest in using such substances is greatly diminished, though this finding is not consistent.

But what is there for us chain smokers?

Here we promised much earlier that we would review the available medical options for nicotine or smoking cravings. As most laypeople appreciate, this is one of the most challenging and frustrating areas we face as physicians. A practice that is so costly, both from a medical and financial perspective, yet so difficult to curtail or eliminate has led to many sleepless nights on the part of my colleagues. Just as we fervently hope for the development of effective tools in any addictive disorder, we await a more promising tool for smokers. Naturally, those smokers who simply take their chances and accept the repercussions of this habit can be difficult to motivate. If they present their familiarity with the huge body of evidence that should incite them to quit, yet they insist on keeping this vice, we are often at a loss. If they show any willingness to forgo this behavior, we can at least offer some medical means of minimizing their misery and increasing their odds of success. With the most motivated and compliant patients, we have a success rate of about 35 percent, though many of my colleagues who practice hypnosis and offer Smoke Enders programs and other means of facilitating this painful process might offer a more optimistic number. Any patient who remains engaged in treatment—whether behavioral, medication-based, or cognitive—has a considerably higher likelihood of successfully quitting. But, as I mentioned earlier, smokers require an average of seven attempts before they quit for good.

First we have the longstanding approach of nicotine replacement—"the patch"—which has been helpful to a limited extent. This is the approach that we utilize in inpatient units, where the vast majority of patients are temporarily quitting against their will, due to hospital policies. The patch does make patients more comfortable and minimizes the symptoms of withdrawal that would afflict a moderate to heavy smoker. Side effects are modest, as long as the patient removes the nicotine patch prior to sleeping. We can adjust the dosage to accommodate all degrees of smoking, within reason.

The downside is that we are replacing one dependence with another, though the act of applying a patch in the morning is of little consolation to those smokers who eagerly look forward to that first smoke of the day. This approach also requires that the patient cease smoking from day one, which is often unrealistic. Most patients will confide that their craving for a cigarette remains quite intense despite the presence of nicotine. For this reason, the more sophisticated approaches have a higher success rate by virtue of the fact that they diminish the urge to light up rather than merely easing the withdrawal symptoms, which are only one factor in perpetuating this addiction. Medicine currently offers two agents, both of which appear to interrupt the pathway which leads to ongoing craving for cigarettes.

Wellbutrin (aka Zyban) and Chantix

Wellbutrin has been used for over twenty-three years as an antidepressant, with reasonable success. It has a favorable side effect profile and is unlikely to trigger anxiety, insomnia, or tension when started slowly, especially in the slow-release formulation. For marketing reasons the pharmaceutical company that manufactures Wellbutrin has chosen to offer a second tablet for smoking cessation, most likely to avoid confusion and allay fears about the use of an antidepressant. A half dose is usually easily tolerated; though, when a patient complains of side effects, I often note that they are trying to quit cold turkey instead of making use of these safe and often effective tools.

The second option is the medication Chantix, which has now been available for several years. Success rate is about 39 percent, with adverse effects that can include stomach upset, irritability, and nightmares, and possible mood swings. So the patient has to be fairly interactive and responsible in order to ensure safe treatment with this agent.

On a positive note, both of these options are generally well tolerated, and they help to counteract the common weight gain that many ex-smokers experience in the first months of smoke-free living.

Chapter 7

Beyond Medication –
Non-pharmaceutical Treatments

What about diet and exercise? I prefer a holistic approach!

I am always thrilled to hear these questions, since I value nutrition and exercise as an essential part of taking care of oneself. Healthy mind, healthy body, as the expression goes. And there have been many studies of the impact of various dietary supplements on mood and anxiety, including various amino acids, fish oils, vitamins, etc. Unfortunately there have been no convincing results to date. And this appears logical, since the chemistry of the brain is so complex that I would be surprised if a single ingredient could have such a profound impact.

As for exercise, many patients ask about using a regular workout to enhance their level of endorphins or other natural feel-good substances. This again has been researched quite extensively, with promising results for mild anxiety and mood disorders. However, any moderate to severe disorders have not responded to these holistic approaches alone. On top of this, most of my patients have difficulty just opening the mail or making lunch on a daily basis. To ask them to spend two hours in the gym every day or cook a five-course macrobiotic meal would only add to their sense of being pressured and feeling inadequate and overwhelmed. Those of us who are covering all the bases with our lifestyle are in general many steps ahead of the average American. These health nuts are usually immune to the low energy levels, lack of motivation, and inability to focus on, and follow through with, goals that characterize the depressed patient. When a holistic type does develop a depressive disorder, it can get complicated, since they are generally uncomfortable accepting traditional remedies such as medication or therapy.

As for the patient who hopes to benefit from the body's natural opioids, or endorphins, I say more power to you. Even though I try to be reasonably active, I have only experienced the so-called "runner's high" a handful of times in my life.

Behavioral Treatment

So does it matter if I get off the sofa?

Of course it does! Unlike medically compromised individuals, to whom it seems logical to remain in bed and recuperate, the vast majority of my patients deteriorate when they have too much down time. While most depressed patients gravitate toward their bedrooms, the role of treatment is to mobilize them as quickly as possible. Just as we expect a patient with a recent hip replacement to resume walking as soon as possible after his or her surgery, we also push someone with a mood disorder to start functioning again. Initially this could include extremely modest goals. Eat three meals a day. Seek out four human interactions each day. Take some written or mental notes on your feelings, thoughts, and experiences. Keep up with your therapist and doctor on a regular basis. Ask one or more members of your support system to learn more about your condition and assure them that you are working on your recovery. And keep in mind that these goals will get easier with time.

So how do I "de-stress?"

As many of my patients have put it, all they really ask of me is that I help them achieve "inner peace," as if that were available as a capsule, packaged in a large jar sold at Costco. But as Freud explained in an elegant and in this case fairly straightforward paper, the total absence of stress would in fact be quite boring and unpleasant. The goal he described would be to maintain an optimal level of stimulation, not too high or too low, which would motivate us to get off the sofa without driving our blood pressure through the roof.

Many patients with the most extreme form of stress, which psychiatrists have described as a panic attack, have a sense of "impending doom." This tends to trigger a fear of dying, either via cardiac arrest, respiratory failure, or some other acute catastrophe. Once my patients who have suffered through these attacks are able to accept that they are not in mortal danger (often only after several costly and extended visits to the emergency room), the panic attack by necessity has lost much of its impact.

On the other hand, most of us still seek an antidote to these miserable episodes, which largely explains the popularity of such sedatives as Valium, Xanax, and alcohol. Who wants to waste their time breathing into a paper bag, or doing some sort of Eastern breathing exercises? Why not just take advantage of the pharmaceutical industry's offerings as a quick fix? One major problem with this plan is that anxiety is often not limited to these attacks but often consumes many frustrating hours each day. So the use of potent sedatives around the clock becomes quite tempting, though I for one have never cured any of my patients with a large bottle of Valium. In fact, reliance on these medications tends to lead to many adverse and insidious effects, including sedation, amnesia, and even depression, not to mention addiction and higher risk of falls, car accidents, and general underperformance. However, the most pernicious effect is that one is relying on an external agent, rather than building up coping skills and developing relaxation techniques. This approach can also lead to a pattern of ignoring or avoiding problems, rather than addressing them head-on.

What is your game plan for getting through the day when I feel overwhelmed or hopeless?

Following below is an actual plan that I typed up at the end of a session with one of my outpatients. When a doctor meets with a patient, the patient retains only about 20 percent of the material discussed. And when the patient is in distress or for any reason incapable of focusing well, the retained percentage drops considerably lower. So I have often resorted to the use of a written summary, which the patient—and, ideally, one of his or her family members—can take with them in order to have at least a basic comsorder.

Treatment Plan for Steve

1) Stabilizing medication program

2) Nutrition—maintain regular meals as much as possible.

3) Exercise—walking, playing with your dog, going to the gym, mopping kitchen, etc.

4) Maintain communication and basic social interactions.

5) Consider having a family session in the future.

6) Recognize that long-term medical disorders can cause frustration and burnout—both for the patient and his or her loved ones.

7) Try a support group—consider the stress management group in my office.

8) Make use of relaxation exercises, recordings, etc.

9) Keep in mind that mood disorders do improve with consistent effort and time.

As you can surmise, these goals are not overly complex or ambitious at the outset. Most of my patients have become so anxious and fearful that their basic body functions are disrupted. Just getting back to a regular schedule is often the single most important role of treatment in the first phases of recovery. When I worked in the hospital setting, much of what we accomplished revolved around rousting patients from their beds and engaging them as much as possible in basic educational, social, recreational, and physical activities. We also enforced (as much as possible) many rules, which were often the cause of bitter complaints: "Why do I have to take a shower at seven in the morning?" "Why do

I have to go to group therapy?" Why do I have to show up at lunch if I'm not hungry?" The return to a regular routine for a patient who has no clear structure or goals has an enormous impact on his or her sense of control and usually substantially reduces the level of anxiety in short order.

The second principle that is critical to recovery is to seek out support by any means possible. Suburban life in the twenty-first century can be extremely isolating, social networking, speed dating, bar crawling, etc. notwithstanding. In the above case, the patient felt abandoned by his family. They had come to visit him the first seven times he was admitted to the hospital, but he did not understand why they stopped visiting after the seventh admission and why he had been alone for his five most recent inpatient stays. Involving any existing family members who are willing to join in can be extremely effective provided that these individuals are supportive and encouraging and minimally judgmental.

In this patient's favor (though he was an extremely challenging client) were the following strengths:

1) He took the trouble to find a new specialist, despite many frustrating past encounters.

2) He was willing to modify his medication regimen at my discretion.

3) He had maintained ownership of his pet, which was a powerful commitment on his part. This serves to help patients get moving and often deters them from harming themselves, since they worry about their pet's welfare.

Unfortunately he had come to view himself as a victim and tended to focus on his sense of being neglected, rather than making an active effort to engage others in his recovery.

Here's another sample crisis plan, in this case for a patient who was virtually fixated on her marital dissatisfaction rather than embracing her own role in managing her mood disorder:

Treatment Goals for Bonnie and Clyde

1) I deserve to be respected and to be heard.

2) I agree to work on respecting and hearing other people's concerns.

3) I agree to put off major decisions until my mood and stress level are stable.

4) I agree to maintain a healthy life style and work on managing my stress levels.

5) I am willing to work on minimizing conflict and will actively focus on avoiding extended "investigations" or accusations.

6) I will work on setting aside short periods of time to focus on building up my relationship.

7) I will work on minimizing the temptation to blame others for situations that may or may not be under their control.

8) I can maintain a reasonable support system.

9) Consider stress-related groups such as the mental health association, etc.

10) Keep in mind that relationship problems do improve with consistent effort and time.

As you can see, this was complicated, since my patient insisted that her husband accept an active role in the treatment process. We thus formulated a plan that included both of them, with a focus on setting some basic guidelines and avoiding the blame game.

How do I learn to cope in five days or less?

Here I have to give my patients both good and bad news. The good news is that most of my patients have already learned to cope with a variety of difficult situations over the course of their lives and have merely lost confidence or encountered a series of setbacks that have become overwhelming. It is reasonable to remind each of them of their past success in dealing with adversity, and to review the skills that helped them succeed. I also find it helpful to break down their current challenges into more digestible bites. Applying the serenity prayer also goes a long way, in that we usually cease worrying about problems once we recognize that they are beyond our own control.

On the other hand, many of my patients who have been failing to take an active role in managing their problems and who have been essentially sweeping issues under the rug for many years, will ultimately arrive at the point that there is no more room down there. At this point they will eagerly—or angrily—arrive at my office, take a seat with their latte, and attempt to unload ten or twenty or more years of setbacks, disappointments, and complications in the course of a one-hour-long initial session. Naturally they are typically displeased to learn that their time is up and that we will in fact need to set aside considerable time and energy to discuss these concerns and some potential remedies. Not only do we need to compress twenty or more years of setbacks and frustrations into fifty minutes, but then we need to formulate a reason for these misadventures and some potential or even surefire solutions. During my years as an inpatient physician, I had the luxury of at least four or five days for this process, which has now been reduced to a mere hour.

Whether due to the need or desire for a simple explanation, or because of our modern era of genetic and neurochemical progress, my field has largely become quite biological in nature. We like to explain how medical disorders develop in a more scientific manner, rather than returning to Freudian theories or other psychological hypotheses. We rarely speak about defense mechanisms or the intrapsychic (meaning psychological) conflicts that are the root of most anxiety disorders. Most current psychiatric research revolves around genetic or pharmacological applications rather than exploring new forms of therapy. Thus many of my colleagues rely on big Pharma to support their research, teaching, and other academic pursuits. Plus, over the past twenty years, our colleagues in psychology or social work have largely taken our places in the analytic institutes, where psychiatrists had in the past been most invested.

Following the lead of physicians, and certainly of managed care models of treatment, many patients would prefer to view their predicament as the result of a simple chemical imbalance, since this to a large extent takes them off the hook. In addition, based on modern medical interventions, promoted by the relentless pharmaceutical industry as well as many biologically based psychiatrists, many patients appear to believe that abnormal neurochemical processes can be more easily corrected than an unfortunate pattern of exercising poor judgment or struggling with impulse control. But most of my patients ultimately accept that much of their success in their treatment—as well as in their lives—will rely on their ability to make better decisions. They are also humble enough to accept that many challenging situations will call for backup in that they should not take on the world on their own. Plus, a well-adapted individual has the confidence to change course and make changes when indicated. Modifying medication regimens is just one example of this process, which can often be quite intimidating for many patients who harbor a great deal of anxiety about the potential effects of various psychiatric medications.

What sort of activities will boost my mood?

This part becomes more complicated since we all tend to value and benefit from different endeavors, but there are some common themes here, which generally apply to most, if not all, of us.

1) Avoid isolating.

2) Try to include some physical activity in your day. If you notice your dog eagerly waiting by the door, walk him or her. If you don't have a dog, walk yourself. Or borrow the neighbor's dog.

3) If you value spiritual or religious involvement, this is generally very helpful.

4) If you have an affiliation with any specific group or organization, whether your workplace, a club, a support group, etc., it is important to include this group in your recovery—provided that you feel comfortable doing so.

5) Laughter is often the best remedy, though it may seem inappropriate to make light of a frustrating or overwhelming situation. This goes back to the old expression that says, "If I wasn't laughing, I'd be crying." Humor is one of those precious tools that can help us get through a challenging situation, day, or more extended period of time. Often it might take some time to regain this ability. Try to seek out and spend time with others who make you laugh.

On many occasions a helpful approach is to ask my patients to compile a list of their ten favorite activities—or as many as they can come up with. If they are unable to enumerate more than two or three, which is often the unfortunate case, we start to comprehend the basis for their frustration. It is often remarkable how little time most of us set aside to keep up with these interests or passions. I often have to prompt patients to think back to their high school or college days. As adults we often focus primarily on our obligations and responsibilities, and over the years we forget how to take care of ourselves or simply have fun. Even the task of making such a list seems frivolous to many patients, just as my recommendation to plan a vacation, watch a comedy, or sing karaoke (even if it's off pitch, like yours truly) is often greeted with a skeptical "Sure, Doc!" If one is capable of fitting in at least one rewarding activity per week—or, ideally, per day—then one is way ahead of the rat race. As fearful rats who mainly worry about their survival, we are only focused on paying bills, going to work, taking care of other people (generally from a sense of obligation rather than enjoyment), and other nonrecreational endeavors. But what about the payoff for all this hard work? As the old adage tells us, all work and no play makes Jack a dull—and most probably, depressed—boy. And in the past year, I have heard the more modern version of this truism, which points out that he who succeeds in winning the rat race is still a rat.

Here I would have to point out two major concepts related to dealing with stressors. First, most patients who suffer from depression tend to dwell on problems that are entirely beyond their control, while more fortunate individuals let these problems go. Those of you who are familiar with the serenity prayer understand this concept. If we focus mainly on areas that we can change, we will likely be much more successful and better adjusted at the end of the day.

The second principle is that we all react to situations in many diverging ways. Those of us with a more positive reaction will tend to find life more rewarding, while those who tend to panic—or catastrophize, in psychiatric lingo—will generally wish they had stayed in bed. The ability to modify one's reaction is the basis for the field of cognitive therapy. This work tends to take much time and energy, but in the long run it is critical to one's mental health and overall success.

The world is going down the tubes, and there's nothing I can do about it!

This pattern of reacting to the world around us, and more importantly, to ourselves, tends to be quite apparent in my first clinical encounter with a new patient. "My kids don't listen to me." "My neighbor's lawn is greener than mine." "I thought I would be married with two children by the time I was thirty-five." While one could view these as simple complaints based on frustrating situations, I would instead label these as either self-imposed pressures, maladaptive comparisons, or unrealistic expectations. These will all trigger not only anxiety and frustration but also automatic negative thoughts. This is the classical "glass half-empty" viewpoint. My most striking experiences in this arena occurred in the inpatient units, where I worked for fifteen years. Most of our patients came into the unit with the conviction that their lives were worthless and hopeless, but they generally felt entirely different five to ten days later. Naturally not much had in fact changed in that short span of time, during which they were in fact cloistered from their usual pressures and responsibilities. Rather, what occurred during treatment was a potent process by which their perceptions were dramatically altered.

This brings to mind the joke about two men who were facing the same miserable situation. They had been fired, their wives were leaving them, their teenage daughters were pregnant, and their houses were being foreclosed on. The first was found on a bridge, ready to jump off.

One might find this reaction appropriate, at least until encountering the second man, who took this quite different perspective: "I was smarter than my boss, and I have already found a higher-paying job. My wife was a terrible cook, and I'm looking forward to getting back to dating. I always wanted to be a young grandfather and am quite thrilled for my daughter. Finally, I'm glad my home is being foreclosed on, since that means my cantankerous wife will have to find a job and an apartment." So it is how we view the world, rather than how the world is actually treating us, which determines our success at the end of the day.

The most critical issue in this regard is not the external world, but rather our view of ourselves. This was captured in many self-help books from the seventies, such as *I'm OK, You're OK*. The current epidemic of low self-esteem has certainly been a boon to my profession. As the cliché goes, most of us are our own worst critics. We compare ourselves to others, we focus on various regrets and mistakes that we have made in the distant past, and we dwell on our flaws and imperfections, rather than our strengths. Even coming to consult with a psychiatrist often undermines someone's self-esteem, especially when he or she is confronted or labeled with various disorders and character weaknesses. This is why I tend to set aside some time even in the first visit to emphasize the patent's strengths and past successes. I also emphasize that the vast majority of patients improve with time and will learn to manage their sources of stress quite effectively.

What about if I sing when I do the laundry?

This raises the million dollar question. How do we keep having fun as mature adults who have to take on more and more responsibility and pressure as we age? Why is it that children seem to have all the fun and then they grow into stressed and frustrated young adults? This is the reason for all those talk-show guests who exhort us to find our inner child. In the media we appreciate the efforts of Walt Disney to appeal to our children as well as to us, the parents. What do we admire about movies such as *Mary Poppins* or *Mrs. Doubtfire*? What about songs such as "Whistle While You Work"? These are all examples of making lemonade out of lemons. Anyone who can transform menial household tasks into rewarding and joyous occasions would clearly make a good therapist, or a good companion, for that matter. These tasks, which we refer to as mastery activities, may not be the highlight of our day, but they allow us to enjoy life by laying the foundation for success. Though paying bills, cleaning the kitchen floor, and making a healthy dinner are not glamorous events, the alternative is much worse. Those of us who neglect these tasks tend to struggle with other areas. Think of the ant and the grasshopper. The grasshopper, who played all summer, complained of hunger once winter arrived, with an unreasonable expectation that the ant would bail him out. I generally advise patients to use these principles when they contemplate distasteful chores or obligations:

1) Set aside limited periods of time so that the chore does not become overly onerous and then move on to a more rewarding endeavor.

2) Try to include others in these events if possible so that this becomes a social interaction.

3) Remind yourself that you are managing your environment in order to have more success getting what you want and need.

4) Reward yourself regularly for your efforts in a meaningful manner. This might include just appreciating the fact that you have a shiny kitchen counter, or that you have no bills to worry about for the next month. I know when I get my cholesterol checked or bring back an overdue library book, I give myself a mental pat on the back and promise myself a dinner out or a trip to the boardwalk.

But I just have too much on my plate to have fun!

Here again, it is often difficult to view life's many pressures as challenges that allow us to use our skills and build our confidence. But I would submit that most activities that we view as chores are not intrinsically distressing if we are able to view them in a more positive light. As many self-help experts suggest, turn on your favorite soundtrack. Invite a friend or relative to help out in return for a home-cooked dinner (or a trip to the movies for those who don't find cooking enjoyable).

Using Your Mind in Your Favor—the Power of Positive Thinking, or Cognitive Therapy

How do I keep it positive?

Of course, most of us would prefer to see the world and ourselves with rose-colored glasses. Some key principles here include focusing on the present rather than the past or the future, since only the present is potentially under our control. This indicates the benefit of shifting the focus away from various past wrongs or slights, though this can be a challenging process. Another goal is to avoid unfair comparisons and to take into consideration our past obstacles and challenges when assessing our level of achievement. It is also often worthwhile to revisit a patient's definition of success. Is one's worth measured by one's bank account or by the size of one's home? Is it based on one's position on the corporate ladder, which can be quite treacherous? Does it rely on our spouse's approval and our children's ability to make the dean's list every semester? In addition, we often focus on our mistakes or past errors. I tend to use the at times painful example of academic testing, in my past years of college and medical training. When I received a grade of 82, did I reward myself for the forty-one out of fifty items that I answered accurately? No! Naturally my focus immediately shifted to the nine errors, highlighted with red ink, which I misunderstood or otherwise bungled.

In general I do not recall having appreciated the effort expended to be able to respond correctly to forty-one out of fifty items.

So the power of positive thinking is no joke? Why can't I be more positive?

Many studies in which patients are treated with sugar pills also are quite successful. Usually about half of the study patients perk up and have a clear-cut improvement, with no active treatment. This is disconcerting in a way, but it also means that I need not worry as much about my proposed plan of action. Even if I do nothing other than hold the patient's hand, he or she will likely be much improved in the next four to six weeks. This parallels the medical world, in which by example I might take a given antibiotic for my lingering upper respiratory infection. Perhaps it proves ineffective after seventy-two hours, at which point I try a second costly but popular medication. Then, forty-eight hours later, it finally seems to take effect, and my symptoms finally remit. So of course the second medication becomes a family favorite, highly vaunted to all my friends and relatives. "That Z-Pack really did the trick." Our expectations of benefiting from an intervention play a powerful role in how we make sense of the world around us, and of our own well-being.

Of course, I might also give some credit to the chicken soup that—with any luck—my wife prepared for me. Or even just the fact that five days elapsed and my immune system likely took action would be another possibility. But it is human nature that we prefer to take the bull by the horns, even if he is walking in the right direction without our guidance. Why leave anything to chance when those beneficent pharmaceutical companies have a cure for virtually any conceivable ailment, and even some that we haven't yet conceived of?

Why do some people always seem to be having more fun?

This goes back to the old expression, often repeated by one of my favorite supervisors, that "It's better to give the ulcers than to get the ulcers." In my view there are two camps out there—the first, those of us who take the blame for just about any and all problems in the world. If we get downsized, it's because we underperformed and didn't spend enough time in the office over the Christmas holidays. If our spouse seeks a divorce, it must reflect some failing on our part, rather than his or her commitment issues. If our child fails to enroll in a prestigious college, that implies that we didn't help them with their algebra homework or didn't find the resources to fund their education in that overpriced prep school that that irritating neighbor's son attended.

The second camp, of course, is the exact opposite—those of us who are covered in Teflon. If I was fired, that's because the boss's nephew took my job. If my wife decides to seek a divorce, that proves that she's having a midlife crisis and has become hormonally imbalanced due to menopause. If our child did not get into Harvard, that's because the neighbor—whose daughter did get in—plays golf with the admissions officer. Unfortunately for the first group, members of this second group are somewhat immune to stress, in the sense that they will rarely accept any responsibility for problems or setbacks. I don't recommend their approach to coping with life, but at times I will chide those overly responsible types to become a bit more irresponsible. Most setbacks in life are the result of several events, many of which are not under our direct control. So the optimal stance would ideally be somewhere in the middle, where we can respect the words of the serenity prayer. This exhorts us to take responsibility for only those areas under our control, which at the end of the day will lead us to much more success and confidence. This also helps us accept that sometimes we cover all the bases but still get called out at home plate.

How do I stop beating up on myself?

Most of us do have moments - or even extended periods - in which we question ourselves in one or more areas of our life, whether academic, vocational, social, or even recreational. I worked with one patient who had an unusual form of anticipatory anxiety. He dreaded his Sunday morning softball games. Rather than just playing the game, he was virtually paralyzed with fear. Would he strike out to end the game or flub an easy grounder? This fear of failure represents an example of an automatic negative thought. These thoughts are the basis for many cases of anxiety, depression, or otherwise unpleasant mood states. We can't easily eradicate these thoughts, but we can work on managing and replacing them as much as possible. This is a difficult process, since these thoughts are deeply rooted in core beliefs about ourselves that often are triggered by events or setbacks. Once we recognize that these thoughts are often magnified, exaggerated, generalized, or otherwise distorted, we are able to stop making a mountain out of a molehill. It takes practice, since we have been rehearsing these negative thoughts most of our lives. But it's worth it.

What about just thinking positive?

If it were only that easy! Much of the anxiety concerning parenting relates to maximizing your child's self-esteem and helping them develop into happy and functional adults. Unfortunately, this is often challenging and frustrating, even for those of us who are familiar with child development. In spite of the vast number of experts in this field, many children develop into adults who lack confidence, or what you might refer to as a healthy sense of narcissism. In this way they may ultimately fail to prioritize their own needs and wishes. Much of the benefit of seeing a therapist, or even a coach, supervisor, or member of the clergy is that we find support and validation. We learn from these important figures that we are perfectly imperfect, as they say in the twelve-step world, and that we are worthwhile and deserving of happiness. Unfortunately, there are many negative voices that drown out the positive ones. A woman whose family is critical, demanding, and distant will often struggle to maintain her self-esteem. A man who is unemployed for over a year and unable to support his family will also question his value and competence. Since many of us lack assertiveness skills, these situations often deteriorate to the point that the individual will feel inadequate and become clinically depressed or anxious. And in my experience, these patterns can be difficult to reverse. Many negative roles and dynamics have taken root during one's development, and these patterns can be difficult to modify even when one becomes an adult. It's not so simple to shake the impact of those core beliefs and expectations that we all grew up with.

Accentuate the positive!

I often point out that when we turn the key in our car in the morning, we don't generally get especially excited when the motor turns over and starts. Even though the process of internal combustion is quite remarkable, we take this for granted. Of course, on the rare day when we turn the key and nothing happens, that's grounds for anger, frustration, agitation and even panic. It's going to be a miserable day. As humans who evolved in a dangerous world, one in which saber-toothed tigers and wooly mammoths roamed the earth, we were genetically bred to sniff out danger. Only in this way could we survive the harsh conditions back five or six thousand years ago.

So modern-day Homo sapiens has a brain that is programmed to identify danger and take appropriate action. But today's action involves making a trade on the market, or enduring an extended meeting in which our supervisor puts us on the spot or repeatedly throws us under the bus. As I noted before, these are not fight-or-flight situations. So our body pumps out stress hormones, our blood pressure rises, and our brain fires up the danger center. With no physical outlet, we are prone to develop a panic attack, reach for a drink or a smoke, or suffer from a so-called psychosomatic condition such as migraine or peptic ulcer disease.

So why isn't there a vaccine for stress?

As I mentioned earlier, we tend to be our own harshest critics. We look in the mirror and cringe at that new wrinkle on our forehead. We check our bank account balance and wonder whether we'll ever be able to retire. We try to help our children with their homework and realize that we're hopelessly confused (though, after thirty years, how would you expect to recall the past subjunctive tense of the verb "poder"?) So the take-home message is that we usually have distorted views of the world. This means that problems tend to be magnified or otherwise generalized. The first step is to recognize this process and start to correct the distortion. For example, this often comes up when I discuss a new medication with one of my patients. Most patients could expect a response rate to any given antidepressant of about 70 percent. Those terrible side effects that one hears about on the TV commercial will affect one to two percent of all people who take the medication. Those odds seem pretty good to me but often are frightening to an already fearful and vulnerable patient. Of course, I emphasize that my role is not only to maximize the patient's success, but also to manage any side effects that may emerge. Should those not be acceptable, then of course we could move on to another medication, which will ideally lack that adverse effect. The offending medication will be metabolized and become a distant memory in a matter of three to five days.

Managing distorted negative thoughts goes back to one of my mother's favorite sayings—expect the best but prepare for the worst. One could even ask oneself what would be the worst possible outcome of any situation? I often remind my patients that any problem can be fixed, aside from death and taxes. The bottom line is that psychiatric disorders respond to treatment—not like a case of strep throat, which can generally be eradicated with a massive dose of penicillin, but in a way that is more analogous to a chronic illness such as diabetes or hypertension. Naturally, those who make an effort to take an active role in managing these illnesses, in addition to simply taking their prescribed medication regimen, will have a better outcome. Diabetics who follow their nutrition plan, lose weight, and exercise will emerge far healthier that those who are more passive and just commit to taking pills or injecting insulin. Unfortunately it will always be more difficult to modify our lifestyle than to show up for tests or swallow various pharmaceutical products. It also takes more time, which brings us to the next topic.

Doc, I don't have time for relaxation!

This is one of the areas in which psychiatry has to some extent failed. Our society is measurably more stressed out than it was fifty years ago, in spite of medical, economic, and technological revolutions. Just think of all the options that were not available in the first half of the past century. No Valium, no Prozac, no Ambien, and no Internet to double-check on your doctor's recommendations. This has been difficult to explain on many levels. Our standard of living has improved tremendously in the past fifty years, and we enjoy remarkable freedoms and opportunity. We generally have access to health care and education as never before, though of course the cost of accessing these benefits is rising at a rapid clip. On the other hand, many of the institutions that gave us support and structure over the past hundred years have declined to the point that many of us feel ungrounded and have lost a clear sense of our identity and our goals. Such sacred institutions as organized religion, marriage, and government have all been shaken to the core. Our neighborhoods and communities are less cohesive, and our families are geographically and emotionally scattered. Our political leaders are embroiled in conflict and deadlock.

Fortunately for you, the fortunate patient, inner peace can be yours. If you can acknowledge that the world is imperfect but focus on the good stuff, you will achieve success. If you can focus on the benefits of a medication, rather than the inevitable side effects or rare hazards, then the decision to move forward with treatment will be clear-cut. If we note that our mates, friends, or relatives have some flaws, wrinkles, or problems of their own but choose to focus instead on what we hope are their positive intentions, efforts and attributes, we will be in good company. As the good Dr. Freud pointed out, we lack control over many of our thoughts. But, just as we need to expend energy weeding our garden in order to harvest a healthy crop at the end of the season, we can also recognize and eliminate those pesky and distressing negative thoughts.

Why did God invent anxiety?

As Dr. Freud pointed out so eloquently, anxiety exists for a reason. Just as physical pain indicates that we need to focus our attention on our medical health, psychic pain, or anxiety, pushes us to examine our inner workings. Even though in modern-day society much anxiety is "free floating" or random in nature, this was not the case when Homo sapiens was evolving in a dangerous world. Those who were able to summon up courage and fight off predators and endure famines or harsh climate change survived to the next generation. Now that we inhabit a safer world, there is no clear danger that warrants such an intense response. Our sedentary lifestyles do not allow us to metabolize the stress hormones that course through our veins when our bosses openly denigrate our work, our children refuse to make their beds, or our financial institution declines our refinance application. Those of us who exercise, partake in meditation or yoga, or engage in some other form of stress management are better equipped for these sorts of modern-day threats and indignities. The rest of us have a problem that modern psychiatry has struggled to address.

Here again, anxiety is not the enemy. The total absence of anxiety would actually constitute a state of boredom, which in itself is quite unpleasant. On the other hand, unbridled anxiety, which we refer to as a panic attack or fight-or-flight response, is not easily tolerated.

In the absence of an appropriate coping strategy, any person would be hard pressed to avoid such convenient but ultimately maladaptive responses as resorting to drink or drugs. Some people might become angry and abusive toward others, turning their anxiety outward. Others might turn the anxiety inward in the form of stress-mediated medical disorders. Those of us who are more fortunate commonly have three advantages:

1) Using healthy coping skills to defuse the anxiety to a more manageable level

2) Taking on the situation that has triggered the anxiety, assuming that this would be under his or her control

3) Making use of a reasonable network to share the anxiety in a focused and meaningful manner. This is not the "misery loves company" school of thought, but instead the philosophy that "we are all in this together." Phrased in other terms, most of us would prefer to be in the company of peers who are able to make light of adversity, rather than those who seem to bask in their misfortune.

Don't be so darn responsible!

Even though there is an unfortunate but common misconception that depression, addiction disorders, etc. only afflict weak or irresponsible individuals, at least in my own experience, nothing could be farther from the truth. What jumps out at me often is that many patients appear to blame themselves for many situations that are not wholly— or even partially—under their control. One distraught contractor was shocked that he was not able to save his marriage single-handedly, though it was clear that his wife had no interest in working on their relationship and was out the door. Other patients have been distressed by work-related setbacks, in spite of clear evidence that their companies were in dire straits and therefore forced into massive downsizing. Most of my clients have spent many years or decades taking care of their homes, their children, their bills, their work. In the ensuing shuffle, they often lose sight of their own wishes and goals, of what makes them happy. Perhaps it sounds selfish to those of us who share their sense of altruism, but all of us deserve to enjoy life and have fun on a regular basis. Even writing this guide is gratifying, though of course I also hope to enlighten and ideally entertain you, my devoted readers.

This axiom also comes with a caveat. When misfortune strikes, many of those in the opposing camp—that is, those who tend to shirk responsibility—find a scapegoat rather than taking the blame. This can work well in many cases, but taken to the extreme this approach will alienate others around us who are always forced to be the bad guys. In my view a person with an ideal perspective accepts that at times life is just not fair and that those of us who are capable of accepting that news flash and moving on are most fulfilled in the long run. As they say, stuff happens. The world is imperfectly perfect, as they also say in AA. Often those who seem to be trying the hardest aren't rewarded. On the other hand, those of us who were born on third base might mistakenly think that they hit a triple. We can dwell on these injustices or work with the cards that we were dealt. In my estimation, the best revenge is living well. It is often less productive to expend one's energy seeking out and prosecuting the culprit when one finds a puddle of spilled milk than to accept that accidents happen, simply clean up the mess, and move on.

Another very promising current trend strikes me as Eastern in origin - to simply accept life on life's terms. This approach is called acceptance based therapy, or simply mindfulness, in which the individual focuses on simply maintaining a focused awareness of, and accepting without judgment, the range of feelings, thoughts and physical sensations that he or she is experiencing, rather than reacting to or attempting to "fight off" negative experiences.'

Dealing with tough questions, such as "What makes life worth living?"

This area can be treacherous at times. Those patients or individuals who have not found meaning in their personal or work lives have often had painful or abusive childhoods and do not easily trust others, including a well-meaning but naïve therapist. If individuals lack any clear and positive connection to the world that would deter them from ending their lives, that can be trouble. These patients may in fact be at high risk of suicide and do not generally respond to medication interventions or short-term treatment in a traditional inpatient setting. Our generally impatient treatment approaches based on managed care constraints often become frustrated and at times refer these high-risk patients to state hospital settings for "long-term" treatment. This often is quite demoralizing and can even at times validate these patients' perception that the world is an arbitrary and inhospitable place. The vast majority of us, who recognize that life can be challenging but is overall rewarding, tend to have a difficult time appreciating these patients' point of view. Usually with time they come to appreciate that there is value in some area that they can pursue and agree to go on with their difficult but manageable lives.

Chapter 8

Obstacles to Successful Treatment

Doc, you're going to think that I'm crazy!

Most, if not all, the patients who take the time to find my office, schedule an appointment, and accept the fact that they might benefit from a consultation with a professional are by definition not crazy, or in more appropriate terms, psychotic. Any patient who is in touch with his or her possible functional deterioration is clearly showing solid insight and thus is more likely to remain in touch with reality (at times painfully so). Many former patients have confided after several months—or even years—of treatment that they initially concealed significant issues from me for fear that I would either judge them harshly or decide that they were untreatable. This comes down in most cases to a sense of severe insecurity along with anxiety, to the point that one loses confidence in one's ability to function effectively. As a rule this loss of confidence is by no means a reflection of psychosis, but instead a harsh and unforgiving view of oneself in the mirror. My pat response is to point out that the truly psychotic members of our society are the ones who fail to seek help or those who are brought to our hospitals by emergency workers on an involuntary basis.

Seeing a shrink is so embarrassing!

In a world that is so quick to criticize and condemn, it is difficult to establish that treatment is designed to take place in a neutral, judgment-free zone. I understand that my patients are not perfect and that they have at times made poor decisions. Lord knows they have been made aware of this in many painful ways. My experience is that most patients seeking help are not unmotivated slackers who are looking for a practical means of evading responsibility but instead are overly demanding of themselves. Many patients appear to blame themselves for events that were clearly not under their control, such as being served divorce papers by a hostile, critical, and rejecting partner. Or being let go from a struggling company that cannot even make payroll. These feelings of shame and inadequacy can unfortunately be exacerbated by the sense of vulnerability inherent in seeking a psychiatric consultation.

In this vein my first priority is establishing a context for whichever difficulties the patient might bring to the table. This takes place in a supportive and nonjudgmental fashion. I cannot emphasize enough that the majority of patients—whether they come in with mood disorders, addictions or family-based, legal, financial, or vocational setbacks—tend to punish themselves in an exaggerated and protracted manner. Though most of them will require many repeated clarifications of this point, in many cases I can detect a certain degree of relief even from the onset. My usual response is to point out the well-known serenity prayer, which exhorts us to avoid focusing on problems that are not under our control.

Anyone in my shoes would be having a panic attack!

This is a valid point that relates to many of my patients who suffer from what we refer to as a situational depressive disorder. This type of depression is distinguished (somewhat artificially) from a biologically based—or endogenous—episode, in that we can identify clear triggers for the episode. The problem is with this theory is twofold. First, the vast majority of individuals with severe stressors, whether terminal cancer, bankruptcy, homelessness, divorce, etc. do not develop depressive disorders. They of course tend to become sad, stressed and fearful, but remain stable from my perspective. The corollary is that that in the absence of a significant psychiatric condition, most patients would be capable of coping with any given stressor or stressors. By and large, most individuals are remarkably resilient and adaptable. However, the impact of a mood disorder can include fatigue, poor concentration, and feelings of worthlessness, helplessness, hopelessness, and shame or guilt. These symptoms can lead highly successful patients to struggle with even basic tasks, to the extent that they are often trapped in adverse situations. Once they find effective treatment, they can start to modify and improve their circumstances.

As humans we always try to find the rationale for an event, which we attempt to relate in a linear, cause-and-effect relationship. This is occasionally an accurate model, but unfortunately life is generally more complex than that. I find that the biopsychosocial model is much more informative and comprehensive. The brain is quite a resilient organ, just like the liver or the lungs. So any single trigger is not likely to result in a severe depressive, manic, or psychotic episode.

What if I want to tell my boss to jump in a lake, but I'm worried the next boss could be even worse?

This is also quite a reasonable viewpoint. There are certainly times—as I noted in the discussion about medication changes—that one leaves the frying pan only to end up in the fire. It would seem logical that, should this pattern occur repeatedly, an astute individual might decide to stick with the status quo. Based on a series of setbacks and failures, just the idea of any significant change itself would be expected to trigger severe tension and apprehension. Even in many cases in which no clear traumatic experiences can be elicited, many individuals share a pervasive fear of the unknown. We irrationally prefer to remain in a miserable situation, rather than enter uncharted territory. I am often surprised by this reluctance, since in my book change is actually a wonderful opportunity. For those of you out there who disagree, I would present to you the following merits of change:

1) Change offers the potential for making one's life better and more rewarding.

2) Change often eliminates a feeling of being "stuck"—a cardinal feature of many medical conditions, especially depressive

disorders, which are often associated with a feeling that the future is not going to improve.

3) Navigating change successfully can build confidence in your skills both in adapting to a new setting and in making healthy decisions when given the opportunity.

In addition, I would qualify this process by noting that most changes are not etched in stone. In other words, they can often be reversed when necessary. Some cases are more complicated than others, of course. I would not envy the employee who quits her job and then returns a year later with her tail between her legs in search of her former position after a series of unproductive job interviews. Or that hapless male who proudly displays his divorce papers but then realizes two years later that his failed marriage was due to his lying and philandering, and he wishes to reconcile with his distrustful ex-wife. But in general change is a necessary part of development and growth. Those of us who embrace new opportunities tolerate transitions much more easily, which certainly helps in this age of vocational, economic, and interpersonal flux. Since the days of "till death do we part" and cradle-to-grave employment are long gone, we would do well to accept that change is a force for progress, rather than a source of fear.

My family thinks that psychiatrists are quacks!

This unfortunately presents an obstacle in many cases in which one would think that a patient's loved ones would want him or her to have access to the best medical treatment. However, many family members present much resistance to the treatment process and instead offer their own proposed treatment. This can be especially awkward when these frustrating but well-meaning folks show up at the first interview. As a result, we might end up spending the majority of this hour responding to various concerns and protests, rather than using the time to pinpoint the patient's goals and needs. Many self-professed experts in behavioral health will offer their own suggestions, such as making nutritional changes, exercising regularly, seeking out underlying medical concerns, working with a pastor or even a shaman or exorcist, changing jobs, seeking a divorce, etc. Over the course of my twenty-two years in this field, I have seen it all. The good news is that, other than taking away some time from the initial treatment process, these suggestions are often reasonable, as an adjunctive means of helping a patient improve. Who would disagree that we should all exercise regularly, eat healthy food, maintain regular medical checkups, confer with religious figures (for those of us who subscribe to organized religion), and appraise whether our work or marriages are as fulfilling as possible? So of course I would support these measures, provided that they supplement a research-based and clinically proven intervention that I can confidently offer the patient.

For those relatives or friends who attempt to sabotage the treatment process and are not at all willing to tolerate their loved one seeking treatment, I understand their anxiety and frustration. I am happy to answer reasonable questions and include them in the sessions. I do not, however, support their efforts to impede what could ultimately prove to be essential or even life-saving medical care. It is clear that I do not fully comprehend other professions or trades, though of course I might have my own ideas or opinions. However, I would generally possess the wisdom to respect someone's expertise in his or her line of work. For example, if I decide to question the approach that my plumber adopts when he replaces my shower head, I am fully aware that he has the right to bill me for the time that I demand, and also that it is highly unlikely that my wife will allow me to change the shower head in the future, even though I might have paid close attention and taken careful notes on this task.

When I find that treatment requires much additional time and energy due to a multitude of complicated or irrelevant questions, I tend to make use of my policy that any service, either to the patient or to his or her relatives, will be billed if the time involved exceeds fifteen minutes. I rarely enforce this policy, but this has been helpful at times when I find that my phone is constantly ringing, and the communication process appears to be ineffective. Recently I had a poignant example of this process when a chronically anxious and mildly depressed woman came to the office in spite of the vociferous objections of her husband. It emerged that he felt that his wife's overall happiness and fulfillment was his responsibility, and that her low-grade depressive disorder therefore reflected on him as a person and provider. Her medical condition was in his view a commentary on his ability to take care of her. In fact he even referred to himself as a "failure" when it became clear that she was planning to follow through with a consultation. In this case another detail emerged in that the spouse was a first-generation American raised by an Asian family. This brings us to the next potential landmine in seeking treatment.

In my religious/ethnic group we don't believe in formal psychiatric treatment!

As is widely known, many groups do not approach medical or especially psychiatric conditions from a Western perspective. For example, orthodox Jews tend to confer with my colleagues only when their community's concerted efforts to address a behavioral issue have failed. The first line of defense would be their rabbi, rather than a medical doctor. Other groups with this level of resistance include many West Indians, Asians (as noted above), African-Americans, Latinos, and Native Americans. I would generally exclude those of European origin since their attitudes tend to mirror that of Americans. In reality, cultures in relative proximity to Vienna, where psychoanalysis first emerged, tend to be more progressive, just as New York City inhabitants tend to be comfortable with psychiatric care. This likely results from a culture that accepts neurosis, therapy, and Woody Allen films. Alternatively, this comfort level also could relate to the sheer multitude of therapists, analysts, and other mental health practitioners who reside and practice there.

What about special groups—like my grandmother? She wouldn't talk about her feelings in a million years!

As noted in the first chapter, there are many reasons why the elderly are more likely to develop mood or anxiety disorders in their golden years. The challenges they face in this often overlooked period of transition and adjustment can be formidable. The risk of medical illness, loss of a partner, lack of identity with retirement, and limited access to an extended family network all translate into a higher incidence of mental illness. Most of us can deal with almost any pressure, provided that we see the light at the end of the tunnel. When a patient is diagnosed with a chronic illness, such as congestive heart disease, diabetes, or leukemia, however, their expectation is that these conditions are likely to progress and impact their quality of life for an extended period of time, if not indefinitely. In addition, the presence of a chronic pain syndrome is also a high risk for mood setbacks, as you would expect. Finally, the sense of isolation that can accompany one's later years also affects one's morale and can increase the extent of hopeless or helpless feelings.

This population can thus present a high risk of self-injurious behavior and merits close attention, with appropriate interventions called for in many cases. Contrary to popular belief, the golden years may not be quite so immune to mood and anxiety disorders. Part of this vulnerability might reflect chemical changes in the brain, where levels of critical transmitters that regulate our moods might be dwindling. Other risk factors might include a lack of purpose or a sense of being disenfranchised. Still other risks include increasing use of alcohol and mind-altering substances in this population, which is clearly more likely to develop complications from even modest amounts of alcohol that they would have easily tolerated during their college years. So, as you can see, the stressors that might trigger a depressive episode become ever more complex with increasing age. This is the reason that I became very popular with the primary care and geriatric specialists when I offered consultations at a teaching hospital, and an elderly patient suddenly revealed that she was experiencing visual hallucinations of a dog walking on the ceiling. Or in other cases a senior citizen would express suicidal feelings just at their time of discharge, leading to an urgent request for a psychiatric evaluation. Fortunately, most elderly patients are highly compliant and motivated to follow through with recommended treatment, though they do tend to shy away from psychotherapy and often prefer to refer to their antidepressant as a "happy pill" rather than by its name.

What about my teenager? He won't even talk to his own mother!

Now we get to the other end of the spectrum—the young. The above complaint is a common refrain that many well-meaning parents present to my office in a rather frazzled tone. "How do I get my high school senior to do her homework?" "What if my junior is caught at a party drinking and then lies to me about it?" "What should I do if my son drops out of baseball and starts hanging out downtown after school instead?"

The worrisome side to this is that many of these parents are highly competent and effective individuals, but they are somehow incapable of recognizing three basic truths:

1. Our children generally want to be successful but aren't so sure what success even entails.

2. Our children certainly don't want to fast-forward into adulthood and take on their parents' lives, values, and neuroses. (Who could blame them for that?)

3. While teens are not trying to torture their parents, they certainly are not spending the bulk of their day figuring out how to make Mom and Dad happy either. (That's not their job, to be sure.)

Once we recognize these principles, the proper means of managing problematic behavior is more readily apparent. We would benefit from a focus on major expectations and avoid micromanaging. We also need to appreciate that our teens face many pressures and decisions that we thankfully did not encounter one or two generations ago. Life is clearly more complex and more costly as each decade passes. Those of us who feel that our children are unaware of life's pressures are sadly misguided. The fact is that our teens and young people in their twenties are grappling with major pressures, just a few of which I will list here:

1) How will I be able to provide for a family of my own?

2) What do I want to be when I grow up (even though I'm already three inches taller than my father)?

3) How do I keep up with the information explosion and still hold down some sort of job? Do I have enough "friends" on Facebook?

4) Does society offer enough worthy institutions, such as churches, universities, clubs, etc. that are actually deserving of my time, energy, and money? (This is clearly on everyone's mind, especially based on the astronomical sums of money that we are asked to dedicate to our children's educations, with no guarantee of any gainful employment.)

5) How do I avoid becoming demanding, controlling, and neurotic like my parents? They seemed fine until I turned thirteen, but then something terrible happened to them.

Think back to when you were young and self-conscious—weren't you sure that everyone could see that:

1) You had a big pimple on your nose.
2) You clearly gained three pounds over the weekend, or
3) You either got the highest or lowest grade on the math test, either of which is utterly mortifying.

As you can surmise, inviting a teenager to a therapy session can be an exercise in futility. Why would you spill the beans in front of your parents, even if they are paying for the session? No way, José! As they say, the best way to get your teen to talk is to stop asking questions and just listen, though it might take a while.

But I'm going to have to talk about embarrassing stuff!

This can also be a major concern for most—if not all—prospective patients. Even when I reassure them that over the past two decades, I've probably heard it all (though of course in reality I am surprised from time to time), they remain reluctant. Some suggest that they don't want to burden me or that I might judge them harshly. Others simply aren't accustomed to discussing their innermost thoughts and feelings, or to the simply luxury of having the opportunity to talk about themselves in a neutral setting. Still others feel so much shame or guilt that they become overwhelmed and can't even speak fluently for the first several minutes of their session.

Surprisingly, these concerns often subside quite rapidly once we establish that treatment has several rules to minimize problems or concerns:

1) Nothing from treatment is shared with anyone unless this is discussed and explicitly authorized.
2) No judgments are passed and no advice is offered unless it is specifically solicited. Even when a patient directly requests input, this is qualified in the sense that no therapist has a crystal ball, and might offer suggestions that lead to more - rather than fewer - complications.
3) Everyone will be able to move at his or her own pace.
4) Any areas of distress will be addressed at each patient's comfort level.

The only caveat in this setting is a safety concern. If a patient presents a danger to himself or others, we are legally and ethically obligated to take action. In most cases this will lead to an intensive evaluation, either in my office or in the emergency room, with possible referral to a safe setting such as an inpatient unit. So, from a practical perspective, the patient's treatment remains confidential.

For example, if a patient became angry and presents a plan to harm his supervisor, then this would be fully assessed. If the specialist saw any danger to the supervisor, then the patient would be referred to a treatment program. During his stay he would be repeatedly evaluated, and his anger would be addressed and resolved prior to discharge. In this case the patient's homicidal ideation would not be revealed to any individuals outside of the treatment team, so that the supervisor would have no knowledge of this potential threat. Naturally the patient would be referred for ongoing follow-up in order to minimize the possibility of any recurrent angry feelings.

In the less likely scenario in which the patient's anger is not viewed as imminently dangerous, but the treatment provider remains concerned, there is a legal precedent requiring that the intended victim of the patient's plan be notified, in addition to the authorities. This rarely emerges as a treatment issue but would constitute one of the rare situations in which confidentiality might be breached.

What if I lost the family car in Vegas?

Other less dangerous situations, such as marital infidelity, gambling, substance abuse, tax evasion, etc. would all invoke the principle of confidentiality and thus could not be divulged to any individual or authority who was not clearly authorized by a valid release of information. This answers concerns that many patients present regarding their privacy. They wonder whether their health insurance provider will cancel their policy if the underwriters find out about their mood disorder. Or whether their life insurance premium will skyrocket, or whether they might lose their clearance in a high-security position at a bank or security firm.

Are there any circumstances in which my doctor would be compelled to breach confidentiality?

The only situation in which this could actually transpire on a regular basis would be in the case of active military or law enforcement personnel. Naturally, most of my patients would merit careful scrutiny prior to being sent into active combat or traumatic settings. But I would also argue that any individual—with or without established mental health issues—is unlikely to tolerate the stress inherent in a combat setting easily. Should that person be suffering from an undiagnosed and/or untreated mood or anxiety disorder, which is often the case, given the new recruit's common refusal to seek treatment, the risk of an adverse outcome in high-stress settings is clearly immeasurably higher. Most police officers, recruits, intelligence agents, and even public servants are reluctant to seek out and undergo treatment for fear of limiting their career opportunities or otherwise facing stigma. Unfortunately, even physicians and dentists, despite their extensive educations and acute awareness of health concerns, tend to neglect their own emotional health and thus have a significantly higher rate of suicide than the general population. This finding of course would need to be tempered by the fact that the ratio of completed suicides to attempts is much higher for professionals. This reflects the reality that most doctors, dentists, police officers or veterans who attempt suicide generally do so in an effective and lethal manner.

Medication will turn me into a zombie!

This is a common fear that harkens back to the days of Bedlam, or at least to the era of *One Flew over the Cuckoo's Nest*. Was my profession guilty of heavily medicating many patients over the past hundred years, especially in the days in which no safe and effective medications were available to treat severe mood or anxiety disorders? Yes, it certainly was, in many regrettable cases. In fact, much of the work that I focus on – either in my office or in the outpatient programs where I inherit patients who are released from state institutions—is ferreting out which medications are actually pulling their weight and what would be the optimal dose of any given medication. Any excessive sedation or other adverse effect—at times referred to as a "chemical strait jacket"—is not likely to help rehabilitate my patients. Any hope of seeing a patient return to the workforce, help care for his or her family members, or even shave in the mornings, is predicated on helping him or her arrive at an optimal medication program. This will invariably entail some side effects, especially at the onset of treatment. However, most of my outpatients inform me that they have no noticeable side effects after a reasonable period of time, which is usually measured in days or weeks, rather than in months. The generation of medications that came of age during my training years, in the early and mid-nineties, has been remarkably clean in helping to manage serious conditions without a significant downside. In other words, the treatment provided in modern-day psychiatry is certainly not worse than the disease, as many patients fear.

On the same note, I should also reiterate that a medication trial is certainly not a lifetime commitment. Within a period of anywhere from five or six hours to a maximum of four or five days, your liver will successfully filter out and start to break down any ingested substance. If you find that any medication either fails to address the intended problems or is associated with any persistent and troublesome side effect, we simply move on. Unfortunately we do not yet have an Iphone15, a crystal ball, or other diagnostic device that will analyze a given patient's clinical needs and spit out an ideal treatment program. Perhaps someday a smart phone or other technological advancement will replace me. On the other hand, my guess is that it will take many generations of research to synthesize a meaningful set of theories about the chemical and electrical bases for human behavior and pathology.

But I'll become hooked on these drugs!

Many patients have become acutely aware of commonly related accounts of patients who had miserable experiences stopping their treatments. We could all name many celebrities who have had terrible consequences from their use of psychiatric medications. We are bombarded with warnings and cautions about even such benign medications as Paxil, since this can be one of the most difficult to taper and stop. Here it is critical to make three points:

1) Many commonly requested medications are in fact potentially addictive, such as Xanax, Valium, etc. At low doses, however, this is usually not clinically relevant. I invite any patients with this concern to express their preference for a medication program with minimal or no risk of physical or psychological dependence. We also have research that has proven that in the vast majority of cases, newer, nonaddictive medications are more effective in the long term.

2) The belief that one must slowly "wean off" all psychiatric agents has been overemphasized in the past twenty years. While I do not advise patients to stop their medications abruptly, the truth is that there are no major medical dangers in doing so, provided that the medication in question is not a sedative such as Valium or Xanax. Contrary to generally held beliefs, most commonly used medications such as Prozac, Zoloft, Lexapro, and others are not in fact associated with significant withdrawal syndromes. Should a patient on a high dose of Paxil reduce this medication gradually, over a ten- to twenty-day period? Certainly! Is it dangerous to stop rapidly? Not according to our research or my own clinical experience. Could it be uncomfortable in the case of certain short-acting medications, namely Effexor and Paxil? Yes, definitely. These are exceptions, which would be best tapered over a reasonable period of time, with some support from a professional who is versed in this process.

3) Many patients have anxiety about modifying their medication regimen. This can certainly trigger many stress-related symptoms that might be misconstrued as a manifestation of withdrawal, or even as a relapse. I generally advise these patients to allow for some anxiety for a one- to two-week period. If the anxiety persists or increases, then by all means it would be logical to resume the prior medication or a similar one that might prove more effective or better tolerated.

Those patients who are committed to making positive changes or working on their coping skills in a consistent manner with myself or another therapist will generally have more success stopping their medication regimen than those who just cross their fingers and hope for the best. In fact, patients who forgo medication and seek out therapy instead tend to take longer to respond from the outset, but ultimately have a better long-term outcome than those who rely exclusively on a pharmaceutical approach. Those who simply wish to take a pill and have no interest in working on their negative thoughts, expectations, or behaviors tend to find that their anxiety inevitably builds up over the next year or two, with or without ongoing use of medication. So when I am faced with the inevitable question from a patient or their family member: "Do I have to take this for the rest of my life?" I, faithful to my psychoanalytic predecessors, resort to the usual inscrutable nonanswer: "That depends."

I generally ask these folks to choose a relatively calm period in their lives, after they have successfully demonstrated the ability to manage and tolerate stress. Only then do we arrive at a plan to reduce and stop their medication, followed by a final visit to assess their success with this process.

How is this young (actually middle-aged) and unproven physician going to figure out what I should do with my life?

This also revolves around a common misconception about the process of therapy. Many laypeople assume that the patient presents various problems or areas of frustration so that the therapist can present solutions in the form of advice. In actuality, the opposite is true. We are trained to respect each individual's right and prerogative to make his or her own decisions. What do we know? If we tell the patient to leave his or her job, who knows when a better one will come along? If we tell them to sell their Microsoft shares, who knows if their money might have doubled in the next three years? The patient generally has the skills to make the right decision, provided that there is no immediate obstacle to this process. This could include a lack of confidence, difficulty focusing, excessive fear of the unknown or of change, or simply a lack of motivation to make positive changes.

How do I get moving?

This is often the tricky part. We know we have an important mission to take care of but have trouble taking that first step. Most of us are quite responsible, but when it comes to emotional issues, we tend to put things off. "Everyone has bad days," we tell ourselves. "And we all get stressed out sometimes." Perfectly true—I would agree. If our friends or family are telling us that we're almost always irritable, however, or haven't accepted a social invitation in several months, that becomes a more significant issue. In order to move forward, I would view the situation in this way: I appreciate that my support system cares enough to point out the problem. If someone expresses concern about our medical health, we respond in a superficial manner unless we really trust the other person to be nonjudgmental and confidential. If the same person expresses reservations about our behavior, however, we often become defensive and shut down the discussion. There thus appears to be a double standard when it comes to behavioral concerns, whether emotional or addiction-based. This latter category is of course even more treacherous, with most individuals using a heavy dose of denial in addition to their substance or activity of choice. Those who gamble too much are only having a little fun. Those who drink excessively are only "social drinkers," with plenty of good company. Those who like to take frequent doses of painkillers such as Percocet often explain that they have fibromyalgia or other chronic pain syndromes that respond "only" to these narcotics.

Why do I have to hit "rock bottom"?

This old cliché tends to ring true in my everyday practice. Most patients (including yours truly, to be honest) will gladly wait until the sky is falling prior to taking definitive action. Typically, once a crisis exists, then my office phone suddenly starts ringing off the hook. "Can you get me in later today, Doc?" is the popular refrain. Of course this is just human nature. We are so caught up in our everyday routine and activities that it is quite difficult to take the time to set up a consultation. Often I find that a concerned family member or friend —usually female, to an overwhelming extent—actually initiates the treatment process. I am happy to field these calls and evaluate these anxious patients to the best of my ability. Many of them actually expect to walk in within the next hour or so, and they tell me that they have "good insurance" that will cover all but five dollars of their office visit. I find that the availability of crisis centers, emergency rooms, etc. is quite helpful as well. These patients' (or their family members') unrealistic expectations, of course, are a large piece of the puzzle. The treatment process will often shed light on the reasons for their problems, which they tend to attribute to other people's lack of support or poor decisions.

But what about other ways of getting help?

For those of you out there who still do not believe in the science of psychiatry, I welcome you to consider alternate treatment options. While there is a lack of hard data related to holistic therapies, I welcome these approaches as a way of recognizing my well as the value of many of these treatments. Even though traditional Western medicine does not typically recommend or reimburse for these forms of treatment, their value is unquestionable. There are countless approaches that can be helpful, dating back thousands of years to ancient China. At various times in my career, I have suggested herbal therapy, acupuncture, massage therapy, meditation, relaxation, and other means of managing stress-related disorders.

Chapter 9

The Rewards of Psychiatry

Tell me again, why did you go into this confusing field?

This is where we arrive at the so-called happy ending. Unlike many fields that are academically and professionally challenging but deal with difficult and often untreatable disorders, I have the good fortune of being able to treat over 90 percent of my outpatients successfully. Yes, you read that number correctly. Any patient who takes the time to find my office, embark on a course of action, and follow through for a reasonable period of time is highly likely to improve—dramatically. Mood disorders are not chronic illnesses; they usually respond within three to six weeks to an appropriate medication regimen and within three to six months to an effective course of psychotherapy. Do we currently have perfect treatments? No, to be sure. Many patients do find that they are partially better and have to decide—with the help of their treatment team, one hopes—when to reduce or stop treatment. This is akin to managing one's blood pressure or cholesterol, which of course both require ongoing monitoring and possible adjustments over time.

In general, both the patient and his or her family members can readily recognize when he or she is back to normal. Every week or so, I have a patient or two who graduate from treatment and thus reduce the frequency of their visits. Perhaps they choose to follow up with my office every six months or so, or even just as needed. The era of unfocused or misguided therapy that drags on week after week, month after month, and year after year are over. We demand clear-cut and demonstrable results in psychiatry—provided that appropriate treatment is available and that the patient takes an active role in this process.

In addition, as I have described in the sections on biological, behavioral and cognitive approaches to treatment, just as there are many triggers for illness, there are even more ways of managing and ideally curing illness. Most patients whom I evaluate have a good understanding of what helps them adapt to the world and succeed. In most cases they have simply lost confidence, and they benefit immensely from a gentle but persistent reminder that they have already surmounted many challenges and problems over the years. Just as we have an immune system to rid our bodies of infection, with the help of an antibiotic, we have coping skills and defenses for many forms of stress or conflicts. The application of therapy or medication simply supplements the mind's capacity for healing and adaptation.

This talent for adapting is nothing short of remarkable. Most patients who come to my office have assumed heroic degrees of responsibility with little intrinsic reward. Rather than a group of slackers and ne'er-do-wells, the vast majority of my clients tend to take on the weight of the world. For this I give them much credit and admiration, but I also fear for their long-term health. In these cases we focus on sharing the burden, rediscovering recreation and relaxation, and divesting oneself of undue stress. In other words I am able to assume the role of cruise director rather than physician. What about getting back to the basics, before we all discovered work, bills, parenting pressures, yard work, family obligations, etc.? Clearly, all work and no play can make Jack a neurotic and obsessive boy.

I am also fortunate that patients who have decided to seek a consultation are usually prepared to share their most difficult thoughts and feelings. It is a privilege to be trusted with this material, which I value each and every day. Many patients have held onto secrets and fears for several decades, with not a soul aware of their inner struggles, including their closest friends, family, or even spouses. Most of them fear being judged—or perhaps even worse—ignored, dismissed, or patronized. They are vulnerable, authentic, and raw. Fortunately they learn quickly that I am not interested in judging or blaming. Nor am I likely to minimize their fears and pain. I am eager to help relieve them of a heavy burden and also to facilitate any potential change or growth that would lead to a more successful and rewarding adaptation to the world.

Because of this state of inner torment or crisis, many of my patients are motivated and ready to make major changes or commitments. This also sets the stage for the work that generally takes place in the setting of therapy. At times I find myself in the classic role of a physician, who relieves suffering and addresses symptoms. This leaves the process of making changes to the therapist, who often serves a complementary role in the treatment process. I have the option of serving as both treatment planner, medication manager, and therapist, but I often delegate this latter task to a colleague trained in the field, either as a psychologist or a clinical social worker. The former is usually versed in interpersonal or cognitive therapy, while the latter might have an advantage in understanding and treating family systems. The collaboration with a skilled and patient-centered colleague is one of the highlights of my work, especially since most patients benefit from more than one perspective or approach to their problems.

My patients do not present measurable and quantitative disorders, such as elevated blood pressure, serum glucose, or cholesterol. There is usually no interruption of blood flow to the frontal lobe, though the metabolic activity of this lobe is often markedly reduced. I have many approaches or algorithms for understanding and treating various disorders. However, the remarkable fact is that every patient who shares a diagnosis is dramatically different from those who came before or will follow afterward. Each patient I have evaluated over the past twenty-four years is a unique individual, who does not neatly fit into a specific category or diagnosis. This not only keeps me focused on my efforts to understand every patient's unique set of needs and concerns, but also keeps me from resting on my laurels. Each patient has a markedly different set of concerns, needs, and adaptations. This demands a specific and well-designed treatment plan to effect a successful course of therapy.

Ultimately the largest reward for the work that I do is the opportunity to witness the remarkable transformation of a patient who is withdrawn, apathetic, and hopeless into a motivated and enthusiastic member of a family, workplace and community. Those aspects of mental illness that are so troubling—that sense of despair, helplessness, and distress—give way to a new positive outlook and open the door to so much potential and so much fulfillment. If I can share in a small measure in this process of rebirth and redemption, then I am also able to appreciate and rejoice in the process of healing both body and mind.